Praise for *There's No Pill for This*

"My wife lived with MS for fifty years, and her diagnosis started me on the road to holistic health and medicine. I never let her know what her neurologist predicted, and her diagnosis helped me start to teach patients how to live well and cultivate a survivor personality. Dr. Michaël Friedman is what I call a native. He is living the experience; he is not a tourist who doesn't understand—who treats the disease but not the person experiencing it. I truly recommend *There's No Pill for This* because it contains the wisdom of a health care professional who also has the experience of being a patient. Read and learn—participate in your own health and healing and let his wisdom guide you on your journey."

—**BERNIE SIEGEL**, MD, author of *No Endings, Only Beginnings*
and *Love, Medicine & Miracles*

"Though no one wants to partake in trial-by-fire, the experience does, in fact, carve a powerful path and purpose. Dr. Friedman's touching account of the circuitous exploration of his health challenges will help others return to the sacred rhythm of their own lives. He reminds us that we are more than our body and our diagnosis, and offers empowering, insightful, scientifically informed, terrain-based anecdotes and recommendations to address a devastating disease with wisdom and wit."

—**NASHA WINTERS**, ND, FABNO, coauthor of
The Metabolic Approach to Cancer; founder, drnasha.com

"*There's No Pill for This* combines the best of conventional medical treatments with a wide range of complimentary and holistic healing modalities for people with MS. The author, a brilliant and compassionate doctor, has written not only a practical guidebook for both health care professionals and people suffering with MS, but also the inspiring story of his own healing journey. Written with insight, compassion, and humor, this deeply personal book offers hope and direction to all of those suffering from MS and other neurological disorders."

—**ROSEMARY GLADSTAR**, herbalist; author; founder,
Sage Mountain Herbal Retreat Center

"Dr. Michaël Friedman has written the most robust, informative, easily accessible, and helpful book ever for those trying to navigate the rough road of multiple sclerosis. Part personal journey, part modern research, and part clinical pearls, this wonderfully researched guidebook covers a wide variety of conventional, nutritional, and natural therapies as well as novel approaches. I highly recommend this treasure trove of options for patients and their doctors alike."

—**DR. JILL STANSBURY**, ND, author of *Herbal Formularies for Health Professionals*

"Michaël Friedman gives us a clear, genuine, firsthand account of the physical, psychological, and emotional obstacles that MS patients face each day. Through his own experiences, Dr. Friedman has gained immense knowledge and understanding about living with MS, and he uses his wisdom and skills to speak directly to others dealing with such challenges. He lays out the options for therapeutic strategies, weaving in diet, herbs, mindset, nutritional supplements, and many lifestyle activities that can improve the quality of life for MS patients. *There's No Pill for This* is not only for those living with MS, but also for those who live with MS patients, and it will help health providers broaden their perspective and understanding of what their patients must deal with."

—**DR. MARY BOVE**, ND, author of *Encyclopedia of Natural Healing for Children and Infants*

"Michaël Friedman has written the first comprehensive integrative protocol for multiple sclerosis. This book was born out of his fight not only for survival, but also for the right to live a full life with a health condition that can have a terrible prognosis. *There's No Pill for This* is a must-read for clinicians and patients who choose to fight for a better now and a longer tomorrow. Thank you, Dr. Friedman, for bringing your own journey to the public to help others."

—**DR. DECKER WEISS**, NMD, naturopathic cardiologist; founder, Peace Possible

"A unique and powerful personal account of living with MS and using natural strategies to navigate the physical, psychological, and emotional challenges of this mysterious and debilitating condition. *There's No Pill for This* is a helpful guide to empower and offer hope for patients living with MS."

—**AMY BERGER**, MS, CNS, author of *The Alzheimer's Antidote* and *The Stall Slayer*

There's No Pill for This

A Naturopathic Physician's
Personal Prescription for Managing
MULTIPLE SCLEROSIS

Dr. Michaël Friedman, ND

Chelsea Green Publishing
White River Junction, Vermont
London, UK

Project Manager: Alexander Bullett
Editor: Fern Marshall Bradley
Copy Editor: Laura Jorstad
Proofreader: Diane Durrett
Indexer: Shana Milkie
Designer: Melissa Jacobson
Page Layout: Abrah Griggs

Printed in Canada.
First printing October 2020.
10 9 8 7 6 5 4 3 2 1   20 21 22 23 24

Our Commitment to Green Publishing
Chelsea Green sees publishing as a tool for cultural change and ecological stewardship. We strive to align our book manufacturing practices with our editorial mission and to reduce the impact of our business enterprise in the environment. We print our books and catalogs on chlorine-free recycled paper, using vegetable-based inks whenever possible. This book may cost slightly more because it was printed on paper that contains recycled fiber, and we hope you'll agree that it's worth it. *There's No Pill for This* was printed on paper supplied by Marquis that is made of recycled materials and other controlled sources.

Library of Congress Cataloging-in-Publication Data
Names: Friedman, Michaël, 1968- author.
Title: There's no pill for this : a naturopathic physician's personal prescription for managing multiple sclerosis / Dr. Michaël Friedman, ND.
Description: White River Junction, Vermont : Chelsea Green Publishing, [2020] | Includes bibliographical references and index.
Identifiers: LCCN 2020036561 (print) | LCCN 2020036562 (ebook) | ISBN 9781603589727 (paperback) | ISBN 9781603589734 (ebook)
Subjects: LCSH: Multiple sclerosis—Alternative treatment. | Naturopathy.
Classification: LCC RC377 .F75 2020 (print) | LCC RC377 (ebook) | DDC 616.8/34—dc23
LC record available at https://lccn.loc.gov/2020036561
LC ebook record available at https://lccn.loc.gov/2020036562

Chelsea Green Publishing
85 North Main Street, Suite 120
White River Junction, VT 05001

Somerset House
London, UK

www.chelseagreen.com

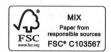

To all the patients who have neurological disease,
and to their loved ones who support them.

Contents

Acknowledgments

My deep gratitude goes to my wife, Sarika Tandon, who has been a great support for me in this journey, along with my very supportive children, family, and friends. I'm also grateful to my healers and neurologists and all the people before me who have had the wisdom to understand the complexity of the body and the powerful healing systems passed down from our global ancestors.

Finally, I'd like to offer a heartfelt thank-you to all my peers who have helped in terms of reviewing, writing, editing, commenting on, and contributing to the design of this book: Jane Dunbar; Gary Miller; Liz Sutherland, ND; Mary Bove, ND; Jen Palmer, ND; Karan Baucom, MD; and Tim Newcomb.

Beyond Pharmaceuticals

*W*hat if you could drastically alter the disease process of multiple sclerosis (MS) using simple lifestyle modifications and restorative medicine approaches that ameliorate symptoms and improve quality of life?

Is this wishful thinking, or reality? Am I chasing the holy grail? Perhaps I am confused about the modern mythology of healing: that almost everything can be cured if you just take a pill, eat the right food, use the right herb, and feel at one with the world. This book is a discovery of my truth in healing.

Sometimes making all the right lifestyle adjustments—avoiding stress, getting enough sleep, developing an exercise routine—isn't enough, and pharmaceuticals are still necessary to best manage MS. On the other hand, restorative medicine—a discipline that assumes a holistic approach to healing using a combination of herbs, hormones, and nutrition to return patients to optimal health—nearly always complements the effects of these pharmaceuticals, and sometimes even outperforms them.

At any rate, as a physician, I know how crucial this question has become in recent years, especially as the rates of multiple sclerosis continue to rise. (Rates of other autoimmune diseases are on the increase, too.) According to the Multiple Sclerosis Foundation, more than 200 new cases are diagnosed each week in the United States.[1] Further, disease prevalence here is among the highest in the world: around 140 cases per 100,000 people in the northern states, compared with the global median of 30 per 100,000.[2] Canada fares even worse: More than 290 out of 100,000 people suffer from the condition. It's a fairly safe bet that you already know someone with this diagnosis. You may even have it yourself.

And it's not an easy condition to live with. Despite the fact that marketing materials for MS drugs always feature a smiling person, the patients I've met aren't that happy. The facts back this up. One recent study found that the suicide rate among MS patients is nearly double that of the general population. And one-third of MS patients have considered taking their own life. Living with an unpredictable and progressive illness can be emotionally challenging and leads to clinical depression—the most severe form—in half of patients.

Whether you or someone you love experiences multiple sclerosis, you or they will almost certainly struggle to manage what are often debilitating muscular and neurological symptoms: weakness in the limbs; clumsiness; double vision or complete vision loss; sensory disturbances; heat intolerance; urinary and bowel incontinence; cognitive deficits such as disordered thinking; and more. While those with MS find a relatively decreased rate of disability progression once they begin taking pharmaceuticals, versus not taking drugs, these therapies typically do not address the root causes of the disease. That's because MS drugs are disease modifiers, not disease treatments. At the end of the day, while drugs do help slow its rate of advancement—and while recent advances mean that some patients can remain symptom-free for long periods of time—MS remains progressive. In other words, just as there's no "cure" for old age (another progressive process), there is truly no pill that can halt MS in its tracks. That's why I chose *There's No Pill for This* as the title of this book: Eventually, every MS patient will face a variety of serious symptoms, whether within the first year of being diagnosed or 20 years later. Everyone will go through the gates of symptoms at some point. MS patients always wonder: *What will my symptoms be?* There is such an array of possibilities. But what particular symptoms will occur will be revealed only as time goes by. Unfortunately, we can't choose, all we can do is try our best, and the rest will be out of our control. I started this book five years ago, and my MS adventure continues.

I have been living with MS for more than two decades. (Although I was not officially diagnosed until 2009, early symptoms suggested I had begun suffering the effects of MS far earlier.) I have learned that living with the disease is complicated. It's often misdiagnosed due to its complexity and also to the way our medical system is structured. It is associated with dozens of nonspecific symptoms. And it impacts almost *every* aspect of a patient's life.

———

Having MS isn't the reason I became a naturopathic physician.* But being a naturopathic physician—who happens to live with MS—is the reason I'm writing this book.

In my dual roles as practitioner and patient, I have experienced first-hand the shortcomings of both conventional and naturopathic medicine in adequately addressing some of MS's most challenging symptoms—and its underlying causes. Doctors know a lot about MS, but the one thing they don't know is how to cure it. My personal experience demonstrates that both conventional and naturopathic approaches can be beneficial, and that drugs or natural supplements can be more or less effective in managing symptoms, depending on the patient and the stage of their illness. And yet many mainstream practitioners are reticent to adopt complementary, holistic treatments: a phenomenon I call "first, do no good" (unless it's standard medical practice).

The core tenet of all medical practice—the Hippocratic oath's "first, do no harm"—has so discouraged health care providers from stepping out of their diagnostic and treatment comfort zones that they often overlook significant opportunities to improve their patients' lives, either with pharmaceuticals or with high doses of herbs. This isn't because of a lack of compassion or desire to provide the highest standard of care with the best possible results. *All* health care providers share a common desire to heal. Rather, I see this as a failure of the system—one that heavily emphasizes specialization (and its attendant compartmentalization) and teaches medical students a formulaic approach to identifying disease through differential diagnosis: "If it's not *A* or *B*, it must be *C*." It also encourages a heavy reliance on treating illness with specific pharmaceuticals for which the risks have been profiled, as opposed to therapies that have shown early benefit, but—most often for lack of research funding—have not yet been subjected to random, double-blind, long-term human trials. Such an ingrained, black-and-white approach means that many

---

* Naturopathic practitioners focus on uncovering and understanding the underlying imbalances that lead to disease, and restoring the body to optimal health using a holistic, personalized treatment plan. This is why, throughout the book, you'll sometimes see me refer to this approach as "restorative medicine."

of today's mainstream physicians simply aren't comfortable with—or practiced in—restorative medicine therapies, including the use of high doses of herbs. But the fact of the matter is that some of these natural approaches are rooted in *thousands* of years of tradition—tradition that modern science is now beginning to affirm, and even improve upon.

If you're a physician, don't be afraid to use the restorative treatments I share in this book. And if you're a patient or family member, don't be afraid to find a doctor who does! As I've learned, restorative medicine can make a significant and measurable difference: ameliorating some of the most troubling symptoms of MS while decreasing its rate of progression.

It's important to remember that conventional pharmaceuticals can effectively slow progression of MS as well. If you're skeptical of drugs, I encourage you to suspend your doubts and try the pharmaceuticals your doctor recommends. Like herbs and other natural approaches, drugs play an important, and at times essential, role in managing the disease. As I've learned to live with MS, I've also learned to hold several truths at once.

This book does not promise a miracle cure for multiple sclerosis; there simply isn't one, at least not today. But it does offer adjunctive treatments and strategies that, when faithfully followed, can delay the disease process and radically improve quality of life. And it's as simple as following a few basic rules of nature to ensure a correctly balanced "ecosystem" for a healthy mind and body.

Although the personal prescriptions I describe in this book are specific to MS, many of the strategies I discuss also apply to a broader range of autoimmune conditions. I encourage you or your loved one to become an active participant in your own care.

CHAPTER 1

Driving on the Wrong Side of the Road

M ultiple sclerosis (MS) is a complex, poorly understood disease that is difficult to diagnose and even more challenging to treat. For starters, many of its physical and cognitive symptoms overlap with those of other conditions such as depression, chronic fatigue, and Lyme disease. And there are four distinct subtypes, each of which progresses (or doesn't) in different ways.

The most common subtype is *relapsing-remitting MS* (RRMS), generally characterized by discrete "attacks" followed by "remission." I hesitate even to use the term *remission*, though, because while patients with RRMS tend not to develop any *new* symptoms during a reprieve, they can still experience serious effects from existing ones. In my own case, I've technically been in remission for five years, but it hasn't been a bed of roses, as I'll share more about later. Remission means only that MRIs (magnetic resonance imaging) of my brain and spinal cord haven't revealed any new lesions (damaged nerves). New lesions means there is new damage to the nervous system. The location of the damage is where the new symptoms will arise. For example, a lesion in an optic nerve will result in double vision or vision loss. In a sense, the idea of MS being "asleep" when a patient is in remission is a fallacy. As new immunosuppressive therapies show, patients who are already in remission still can feel significantly better when they undergo such protocols, which, in general terms, involve oral or infused medications that reduce immune system activity in the hope of blocking the immune system's inflammation and attack on the myelin. The subsequent reduction in existing manifestations of the disease during remission implies that MS is *always* active; how active is simply relative.

The other three subtypes are *primary progressive MS* (PPMS), which is generally characterized by rapidly worsening symptoms and physical function following initial diagnosis; *secondary progressive MS* (SPMS), which often follows an RRMS diagnosis and closely mirrors the PPMS disease process; and *clinically isolated syndrome* (CIS), in which a single physical episode strongly suggests multiple sclerosis, but requires additional evaluation.[1]

When it comes to MS, every patient is unique and can manifest their disease completely differently from somebody else, regardless of the particular subtype they have been diagnosed with. In other words, MS is not an isolated process with a predictable course or a single treatment. In fact, although over 150 years have passed since French neurologist Jean-Martin Charcot first officially described the condition in 1868, there are many things we still don't know about MS. Like how to cure it.[2]

What we do know, however, is that every form of multiple sclerosis shares a common etiology: damage to the myelin sheath that surrounds and insulates nerves, that progresses over time. While no documented cases of MS exist without this, some patients go through much of their lives symptom-free. Their experience suggests that by better understanding this degenerative activity and its causes, we can better address its effects and slow down or perhaps even reverse the course of the disease.

MS Basics

Because I will cover the science of multiple sclerosis more thoroughly in subsequent chapters, I'll just briefly touch on it here. Our brain communicates with the rest of our body—with our arms and legs, lungs and heart, eyes and ears, truly *every* muscle and internal organ—via the central and peripheral nervous systems (CNS and PNS, respectively). The basic building block for these systems is the neuron: a specialized cell that conducts electrical impulses from and to the brain.

Much like any common electrical wire, axons require an insulating layer for optimal performance. And this is where myelin comes in. Known as the brain's white matter, this fatty, protein-rich substance wraps around our axons in a protective sheath, speeding the rate at which nerve impulses can

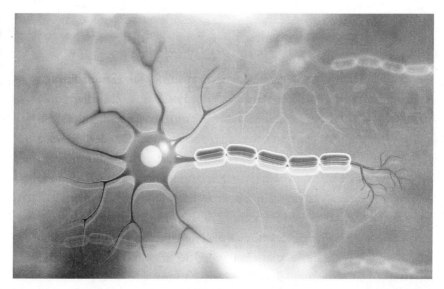

Each neuron has an axon, a long, rope-like structure that *sends* electrical signals from the cell; and a dendrite, a highly branched structure resembling a tree, that *receives* signals into the cell. *iStock.com/Rasi Bhadramani.*

travel along the CNS. For this reason, myelin is absolutely essential for normal physiological functioning.

Premature infants, for example, are very "floppy" in part because their nerves aren't yet fully myelinated. This means that signals from their brains to their muscles don't travel rapidly enough to effect basic physical tasks, such as holding the head upright. Also, because the lungs are underdeveloped, less oxygen reaches the brains of these infants, which interferes with normal myelin production there. Without this essential coating, brain cells can atrophy, leaving these babies more susceptible to neurological diseases like cerebral palsy and even death. In the worst cases, this lack of sufficient myelin can cause significant morbidity and mortality among premature infants.

In addition to oxygen, myelin requires thyroid hormone in order to develop properly. Congenital iodine deficiency syndrome, also known as *cretinism*, provides a dramatic illustration of what can happen when this hormone is absent. The syndrome is marked by severe neurological impairment, among other physical attributes, and it affects children born to mothers who suffered from hypothyroidism and iodine deficiency while pregnant.

When myelin is damaged, whether through autoimmune disease, inflammation, compression, viral infection, stroke, or other causes, nerves can't conduct signals as quickly or effectively as they should. In multiple sclerosis specifically, this damage—*demyelination*—can be so severe as to form scar tissue around the axons, which slows, and in some cases completely halts, the brain's ability to communicate with the rest of the body. As a result patients might experience a whole constellation of symptoms—weakness, fatigue, cognitive deficits, and physical and emotional impairments—that can range from mild to completely debilitating.

In patients with clinically isolated syndrome and relapsing-remitting MS, especially, such symptoms can be nonspecific, variable, and intermittent enough as to make it almost impossible for health care practitioners to diagnose based on clinical presentation alone. But multiple sclerosis is easy to spot on an MRI: Its characteristic scars, or lesions, are visible as white spots in the brain.

MRIs are immensely valuable, both for identifying multiple sclerosis and for explaining its symptoms. However, they don't always uncover new lesions, and they can't be used to track activity in the gray matter of the brain, which includes areas responsible for muscle control, sensory perception, and executive functioning. (Executive functioning comprises a set of cognitive processes that monitor and control behaviors and skills including attention span, task management and follow-through, impulsivity, and working memory.) Additionally, as I mentioned above, doctors cannot use MRIs to predict the course of any particular patient's disease. Some people can live in remission for decades, barely affected by their condition; others might be in a wheelchair within weeks of their first onset of symptoms, blind within months, and, in very rare instances, dead within a few short years. Fortunately, most MS patients are able to be mobile, live fairly well, and still work.

There's no pill for this. Not yet, anyway.

That's the bad news. The good news is that, thanks to pharmaceutical advancements, some forms of MS *are* more treatable now than ever before. Although long-term studies of MS patients remain surprisingly inconclusive regarding the relationship between particular drug therapies and the onset of disability over time, neurologists specializing in MS have noted significant decreases in the rates of disease progression thanks to new treatment protocols. There are more potential therapies for MS treatment and management

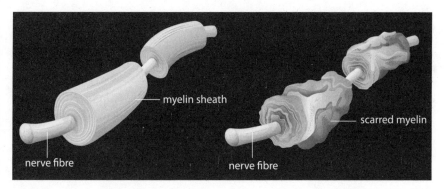

When myelin is damaged by MS, electrical impulses can't efficiently travel via the neurons, which negatively impacts nerve function. *iStock/blueringmedia.*

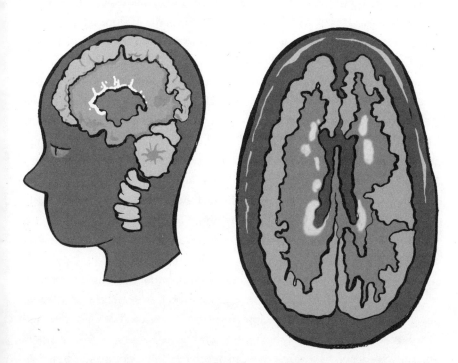

This representation of an MRI of a 40-year-old male (also known as me) reveals lesions in four specific areas: the right lateral medulla oblongata, which regulates breathing, cardiac function, swallowing, and digestion; the pons, or upper medulla, which also regulates breathing as well as balance; the bilateral periventricular white matter (found on both sides of the brain), where axons are concentrated; and along the deep veins in the medulla. These last, commonly called Dawson's fingers, are a classic sign of MS.[3]

in development at the time of writing this book than ever before. In several separate trials, for instance, intravenous rituximab—a drug used to treat rheumatoid arthritis and some lymphomas—has dramatically decreased the cumulative probability of new, or additional, disability among RRMS patients—7.6 percent over a three-month period, with 80 percent remaining attack-free for two years. This drug is now remade and patented as the MS-specific drug ocrelizumab (Ocrevus). Ocrevus has also reduced disability not only in RRMS but also among PPMS patients to 32 percent over a three-month period as compared with 39 percent among those treated with placebo.

Initially, these numbers didn't seem good enough to me—especially for a treatment that can cost upward of $60,000 *each time* it's administered. But as the saying goes, everything is relative, and for those patients who successfully avoid an attack, Ocrevus makes a world of difference. That alone is justification enough for the expense. On the flip side, unfortunately, Ocrevus doesn't only suppress some symptoms of MS; it also indiscriminately suppresses a patient's B cells, a type of white blood cell that produces antibodies that protect against cancer and all infections including COVID-19. (Surprisingly, patients taking Ocrevus anecdotally have fared okay with COVID-19, as of the time of this writing.) Ocrevus has also been implicated in a small but statistically significant increase in breast cancer risk, as well as potentially fatal brain infection.

As I mentioned, it's important to note that such therapies are not curative. They can modify the *course* of MS, but the disease is still progressively degenerative. In an era when so many other conditions *can* be cured with drugs, the lack of a cure can be a depressing realization for those living with MS—and for their families, too.

As mainstream treatments have improved, so, too, has our understanding of the pathophysiology of the disease. Today researchers and health care practitioners alike better appreciate the impacts—both positive and negative—of diet, nutrition, hormones, and other factors on the neurodegenerative process. As a result, we can approach therapeutic goals in a new light: Together with conventional, drug-based protocols, we can incorporate complementary treatments that can both decrease the rate of progression *and* stimulate neuronal health and neuroprotection.

Which brings me back to why I'm writing this book. Those MRI scans I described above? They're mine. I live with MS every day. First diagnosed in my early 40s, I possessed many of the characteristics of a poorer prognosis: I was male, with a brain stem lesion, and I experienced fairly significant symptoms within the first year. Happily, nearly 10 years later I am able to function relatively well most of the time. People who don't know me well don't even realize that anything is wrong. I wrote some sections of this book, for example, while enjoying a cup of tea after a hard day's skiing on Vermont's double-diamond slopes.

Seven years ago, my MS neurologist told me that drugs alone could not explain how well I was doing living with MS, and she wanted to know what I was doing to have such good quality of life. As someone who has experienced remarkable results through complementary therapies, I wanted to share my successes through this book—and I have. But I also need to be transparent and real and share my challenges, too.

My MS Story

My "official" journey with MS began in 2009—although, looking back, it's now clear to me that this disease began to manifest decades earlier in a series of seemingly unrelated symptoms that make sense only in retrospect.

By my mid-20s I had already been hospitalized for episodes of unexplained mental confusion and vomiting. In one of those instances, I was driving a school bus and forgot how to operate the controls. Fortunately, no one was hurt—unless you consider the mailbox I knocked over as I struggled to recall how and where to drive. Despite my explanation of the mental confusion I'd experienced, my doctor concluded that I'd suffered a bout of food poisoning, and he sent me to the hospital for a week.

A decade later I began suffering persistent urinary frequency. I consulted both an acupuncturist and a urologist, neither of whom offered an effective treatment. I realize now why they couldn't help me: Neither understood that the issue was neurogenic—meaning that it was caused by dysfunction in the nerves or nervous system—rather than an infection.

During the months that followed, I suffered from sporadic, yet profound, fatigue. I was also attending the Canadian College of Naturopathic Medicine in Toronto at the time; certainly, I told myself, the demands of the program could have been taking a toll on my physical health. Perhaps, with enough rest, I could heal up and move on. Even though I slept for 10 hours each night, however, I still required daily two-hour naps. On top of that, I had suddenly developed unexplained chemical sensitivities. When the family doctor I consulted told me they were due to psychological problems, I realized I needed to seek answers elsewhere.

That quest led me around the world, from traditional Shuar healers in Ecuador to Ayurvedic practitioners in India. As I broadened my own learning and knowledge as a naturopathic physician-in-training, I also sought alternative treatments for my urinary symptoms (which, I would eventually learn, were manifestations of undiagnosed MS). In Xi'an, China, I checked into an acupuncture clinic that boasted a 95 percent cure rate for urological issues. I spent a ridiculous amount of money to no avail. My Chinese medical doctor, who accepted only US dollars from his medical tourists, once called me "American Dollar" instead of "American Doctor," an apt Freudian slip. In Baja California I went to an alternative medicine hospital where—despite physicians' claims to the contrary—the intravenous "detox" therapies actually *worsened* my symptoms, caused my liver enzymes to spike, and cost

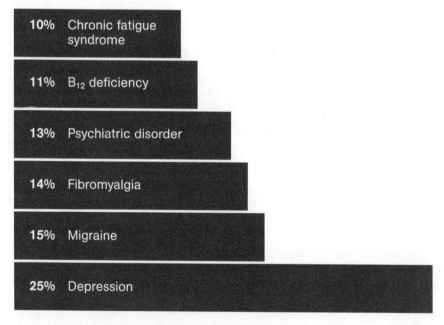

10% Chronic fatigue syndrome

11% B$_{12}$ deficiency

13% Psychiatric disorder

14% Fibromyalgia

15% Migraine

25% Depression

Many MS patients (in 2017, 42 percent) are initially misdiagnosed with another condition. *Adapted from MultipleSclerosis.net.*

$8,000. This hospital subsequently shut down after officials learned that the "doctor" who owned it had faked his naturopathic medical degree and had adulterated his herbs with drugs. These experiences were a hard lesson for me that some unscrupulous doctors do prey on patients looking for the holy grail who are desperate for a cure and willing to pay extravagantly for it.

I also began experiencing intermittent, sharp jolts in my neck when I turned my head. Again, there seemed to be a good reason: I had been involved in a minor car accident not long before, and my family doctor said it made sense that I would experience some musculoskeletal aftereffects. Because neither he nor any other practitioner seemed able to assemble the pieces of my unique symptomatic puzzle into a complete clinical picture, I reluctantly tried to convince myself that I was just different from all of my friends my age.

Then, when I was 40, I suffered a particularly intense back spasm that lasted several days. I'd moved a heavy piece of equipment several months prior, so it was easy (once again) for me to justify this symptom—especially once it dissipated. Except that the painful jolts in my neck and spine returned, becoming so severe that I had trouble with the simple act of eating: Bending my neck toward my plate resulted in electric shocks of pain I felt down to my toes. So I sought help from a chiropractor, who diagnosed me with "overfiring signals." Her treatments, including gentle massage, also provided no relief. As you might imagine, I was becoming increasingly frustrated—and discouraged—by my situation and inability to control it: an unsettling feeling for a naturally upbeat person like me whose first instinct is to find the humor in things. None of this was particularly funny.

A month later, while my wife, Sarika, and I were driving to a friend's house, Sarika asked me a strange question. "Michaël," she said, "why are you driving on the wrong side of the road?"

I realized that I had *no idea*. No idea why I was doing it, and worse, no idea *which* side of the road was actually the correct one to drive on. That frightening episode finally led me to consult a neurologist. He initially thought my symptoms were anxiety-related; surely I was much too young to be experiencing the kind of cognitive impairment most usually associated with Alzheimer's disease or other dementia. Nonetheless, he ordered an MRI, and the results provided the answer to Sarika's question. I'd been driving on the wrong side of the road because I had multiple sclerosis.

The Importance of Persistence

During my first appointment with a general neurologist, he informed me that my symptoms were "impossible" for someone my age. "It's anxiety," he said—but I knew it wasn't. How could he simply write off my complaints? I wondered. Why didn't he believe me? Then I remembered some of my own experiences when I was the one talking to a patient seated on the examining table—and I realized that the blame for the doctor's attitude lay within the system itself.

About 20 years ago my practice included many patients who suffered from chronic fatigue syndrome. These patients had sought my expertise after being told (as I had) that their symptoms were "all in their heads." These patients were grateful that someone finally believed their symptoms were real. Unfortunately, their insurance companies didn't. Unless submitted by a psychiatrist, any claims for office visits related to chronic fatigue were categorically denied. Of course, this reinforced the idea among mainstream physicians that chronic fatigue was a psychological, not physical, issue.

Things have improved dramatically since then, but it's still easy for patients to doubt their own symptoms, and for doctors to dismiss them. This is why it's vitally important for patients to *advocate for themselves*—and for practitioners to listen with an open mind. Such partnerships are what lead to accurate diagnosis and a mutually agreed-upon treatment plan.

Huh? *What?* Neither of us expected this news.

According to the MS neurologist (a neurologist who specializes in MS), the MRI showed multiple lesions in my brain and upper cervical spine and reflected years, or even *decades*, of attacks. Suddenly all of the odd, unexplained, and seemingly discrete episodes I had experienced—the profound fatigue, the shooting pains in my neck, the urinary issues, the mental confusion —made sense.

During the first six months following my diagnosis, I worked with three different neurologists because, unfortunately, the first two neurologists died. My second MS neurologist read my MRI like an astrologer would read my astrology chart or do a palm reading. She said that I probably sometimes get confused trying to figure out the right words to use, sometimes my leg might collapse, my hand probably hurts, and that sometimes I have a hard time censoring my thoughts. Based on my MRI, she could see which parts of my brain or spinal cord were damaged and thus predict what symptoms I was experiencing. So after all, it wasn't *all* in my head; my symptoms were real. And ironically, they were actually almost *all* in my head (the brain).

I asked the first of my three MS neurologists three things. First: What's my prognosis? Second: How will medicine help? And third: Is there anything else I can do?

He told me my symptoms would get worse, but assured me of a good prognosis because medication could slow progression of the disease. He also said that, if needed, he could refer me to an array of therapists—speech, occupational, psychosocial—to assist me in adjusting to life with MS.

With a confidence borne of naïveté, I was certain I would never need this sort of help. Thinking positively seemed empowering. I expected that I could, and would, get better. But mainstream medicine advised me that it would be better to prepare myself psychologically for the realistic probability that my disease would progress. Indeed, this is the advice given to patients with any neurodegenerative disease, including Alzheimer's or Parkinson's.

The National Multiple Sclerosis Society agrees—advising, in its literature, that *managing* the disease, and your expectations for its inevitable progression, is healthier than hoping it will get better. The latter can lead to long-term depression, which does nothing to ameliorate symptoms or a patient's ability to cope.

I wasn't ready to hear this, either. And so, when I received an unsolicited brochure for Social Security disability benefits in the mail a few weeks later, I threw it in the trash.

In the midst of sorting through how to respond to my diagnosis with MS, a revelation came to me: As a naturopathic physician, I *did* know what I could do. I already possessed an effective tool kit for treating patients who have autoimmune thyroid diseases. Since MS is also an autoimmune disease, I reasoned, why not apply those same treatment modalities to myself?

Early Lessons

As it turned out, I *was wrong* and I *did* need help from the specialists my doctor recommended. And once again I was wrong: The specialists were very helpful.

- Occupational therapists taught me better ways to tie my shoes.
- Speech therapists taught me how to breathe and enunciate so I could be understood.
- Physical therapists helped me learn how to prevent my legs from collapsing beneath me.

Since then, experiencing the valuable help such therapists can provide has led me to adopt a philosophy toward life in which I expect nothing, and accept everything.

And so I set out to prove my doctor wrong. I was going to find the holy grail, and I hoped it was possibly right in my lap. I refused to write myself into a script with only one story line: that everyone with MS gets worse. In my mind the process of "healing" is far more nuanced than a series of statistics and probabilities. Rather than starting to take the drug my neurologist recommended, I first decided to follow my father's example. A member of the US Army 10th Mountain Division—an elite unit trained to fight under extreme arctic conditions—my father learned during World War II that the answer to any physical or emotional ailment was discipline and exercise. Since healthy physical activity is fundamental to a naturopath's philosophy and treatment approach, this made sense to me—and the idea of testing my mental and physical grit not only sounded exhilarating and empowering, but also seemed a plausible method for staving off declines in both areas. I signed up for survival training school in the woods of Vermont, where I learned to frame a shelter out of twigs and branches and make a sleeping bag out of leaves. But I ended up freezing, exhausted, and confused about how I could adequately take care of myself in the wilderness when I was suffering from

MS. Despite what I desperately wanted, I realized that my body wasn't up to the task, and after two weeks I called it quits. Admitting to myself that what had worked for my father was not going to cure my disease, I decided instead that maybe restorative medicine could.

I started weekly sessions with an acupuncturist; attended an Ayurvedic clinic where I was massaged with oils (that did feel good!); and consulted a naturopathic physician who prescribed vitamin D_3, a hypoallergenic diet, and the Swank diet for multiple sclerosis, an extremely low-fat regimen pioneered by the late neurologist Dr. Roy Swank. With full enthusiasm and confidence, I tried it all. I just knew that my story line would be different.

And yet during the next three months, my symptoms progressed, and I found myself more fatigued and confused. Merely walking across the living room sapped my energy and strength. A second MRI showed eight new lesions in my brain. Within 12 months I had difficulty urinating, struggled to move my hands, and had to protect them even from benign stimuli like warm water—which would send searing pain up my spine. Playing the piano, one of my favorite activities, was now out of the question. Just tying my shoes took several minutes each—and sometimes more.

I returned to my neurologist; another set of MRIs revealed a significant new lesion on my cervical spine. I felt like I had failed. Was it because I had eaten cookies a few weeks ago? Was I not mentally strong enough to fight the disease? What kind of naturopath was I? I played a list of questions over and over in my mind. I was wrong once again. I did not have the holy grail.

I began a regimen of daily Copaxone (glatiramer acetate) injections, often the first line of defense in MS because it has few side effects, to help decrease the impact of future attacks. But my symptoms continued. My ability to communicate had also been affected—when friends and loved ones spoke to me, it sounded like a heap of nonsense. And when I tried to speak myself, the mental effort was as challenging as solving a complex physics formula. I felt it wasn't worth the struggle, and socializing became stressful. I had failed in my goal to prove my neurologist wrong. Because my knowledge of MS was limited, I didn't possess all the tools I needed to conquer my disease on my own.

Meanwhile, other new and unusual things started happening. I heard sounds that weren't real and conversations that had ended an hour ago. Sometimes those phantom conversations would lead me to get out of the shower in

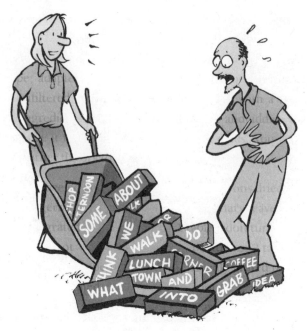

When my MS causes my mental processing speed to slow down, this is how I feel when I try to understand someone talking, even if they are speaking at normal speed. My basic intelligence doesn't change, but the change in processing speed may make me appear to "act stupid."

an attempt to greet a visitor who wasn't really there. I didn't feel pain when I should have, like the time I burned myself on our woodstove; and I *did* feel pain when I shouldn't have, which is a symptom called *paresthesia*. I saw people and objects in duplicate and triplicate—sometimes even tenfold—and it required intense effort to determine which of those images was real. I experienced something called the *pseudobulbar affect*—a condition that causes uncontrolled laughing or crying. I suffered from *time agnosia*, in which the sequence of time didn't make sense; long intervals seemed much shorter to me than they actually were, and I had trouble estimating the duration of short spans of time.

Another time, I entered a café where I ordered a cup of coffee, paid for it, and drank it—but I then needed to ask the barista whether I had already done any of those things. When I was drinking the coffee, my mind thought I was buying it; when I was buying it, my mind thought I was just entering the café. And ironically, the reason I'd decided to have a cup of coffee in the first place is

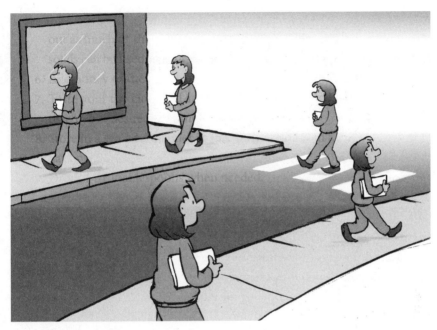

Once, while driving at night, I witnessed the impossible circumstance of seeing the same person simultaneously walking along a sidewalk, crossing the road, reaching the other side of the street, and walking along the opposite sidewalk. This was a manifestation of time agnosia.

that it sometimes helped me feel mentally sharper. I didn't want to tell anyone about these incidents, because I believed they would make me sound crazy.

It often required intense effort and concentration for me to confirm the identity of a person who was sitting beside me. This was true even for members of my own family. For instance, one day I was sitting with my son on our back deck, and I found myself lost in the exercise of trying to distinguish the difference between a son and a godson. Which was he? This became even more complicated as, watching clouds drift over the hills, I believed I was witnessing an active volcano belch smoke over the Andes Mountains. These occurrences of mental confusion led me to worry that I was developing dementia—at age 45! My neurologist diagnosed me with "cognitive decline." I supposed that sounded slightly better.

In a particularly "interesting" episode, I once discovered myself alone in the middle of Burlington, Vermont's largest city, unable to recall who I was, why I was there, whom to call for help, or even how to dial a telephone. It was winter, and I should have been concerned for my safety amid the snow and freezing temperatures—but my cognition was affected in such a way that I didn't have that response. I didn't perceive my situation as a problem. Liberated from my identity, I hadn't a care in the world; nothing I did mattered! An hour later, however, I regained some awareness and realized the magnitude of my situation. I *should* know who I was, even though I still didn't; and when I began to wonder whether my amnesia would be permanent, I felt the full emotional impact of what was happening.

Fortunately, I was able to recall that my neurologist worked at a hospital a block away, so I decided to walk there to seek some answers. When I arrived, I could recall that his office was on the second floor and that I would need the elevator to take me there. Unfortunately, I couldn't organize my thoughts well enough to execute the simple actions required to ride the elevator, like first pressing the call button and then entering the car when it arrived.

Witnessing my obvious confusion, a police officer approached to inquire whether I needed help. I was far too embarrassed to admit that I did. Instead of asking him to assist me with the elevator or accompany me to the neurologist's office, I left. I walked to a sushi restaurant and ordered some food.

I know this may sound unbelievable, but at the time, this seemed an entirely reasonable choice. For me, the cognitive symptoms of MS are so unpredictable and fluid that this kind of perceptual flux can happen at any time, with no warning. In this particular case, once I stepped out of the restaurant, I had remembered who I was. I was back to "reality."

Such rapid progression of my disease made me reevaluate what was truly important. The experiences I'd been having demonstrated that my daily words, thoughts, and steps were limited, and that I needed to ration them wisely. I was forced to consider some drastic questions.

If I could walk only 10 steps, where would I go?
If I could speak only 20 words, what would I say—and to whom?
If I could trust my memory for only two hours, what would I do?

I realized that I wanted—*needed*—more answers.

And so, like many people facing the unknowns that come with serious illness, I educated myself. During the next 10 years, I would learn everything I could about MS from a medical perspective: what it is, what causes it, and how it is treated—both conventionally and using the restorative approaches of naturopathic medicine. Integrating my own professional knowledge of autoimmune disorders with what I discovered about neurodegenerative diseases, I wondered whether certain herbs and supplements I was already quite familiar with might very well apply to MS and yield positive results. So I began to assemble a naturopathic tool kit for treating my disease. In doing so, I began to feel hopeful for the first time in years.

While I was actively educating myself on MS, MS turned out to be a valuable teacher, too. Research indicates that on average, humans have over 60,000 thoughts per day and walk over 4,000 steps a day. With nerve signals being weakened, people with MS can't reach the average for most activities. It's time to prioritize. MS attacks our fundamental identity as a person and what we can and can't do. Of all the emotional and physical aspects that change in MS, the one thing I can hold on to is my values of what is most important, values such as being honest and generous.

By forcing me to slow down, MS taught me where and how I was wasting energy in relationships and situations. By turning my life upside down, it made me understand the fragility and impermanence of life. By making my existence worse when I thought things were fine, and better when I thought they would get worse, it showed me the false nature of expectations. And by altering my perception of sequential thought, it led me to experience human consciousness differently than other people my age—really, most other human beings—did.

Fortunately, my challenges were transitory for the most part, as the episode above illustrates. When I struggled with language, I would remind myself that I would soon be capable of enjoying a satisfying, productive, and "normal" life once again. In the meantime I would play a game with myself, pretending I was preparing for the reading comprehension section of the college entrance exam. Still, keeping up with pronouns while listening to other people talking or reading a story sometimes felt as impossible to me as trying to get a glass of water would be for a child not tall enough to reach the kitchen faucet. At times, I felt I was better able to communicate with animals

Surfing the Waves of MS

One of the most important lessons MS has taught me is the same one that novice surfers learn: You have to ride the waves, not fight them.

Living with this disease, I discovered, is like being out on the open ocean with your longboard. Some days you'll ride great waves; other days you'll crash; and still others you'll face a wall of water so imposing and powerful that you'll doubt your ability to persevere. You'll even have days when all three happen at once.

When I first took up surfing, I wanted to ride every wave that I could. Fortunately, it didn't take too many humbling experiences of nose-diving off my board, or "going over the falls," to discover that I didn't yet have the balance or proper technique to even attempt it. Once I accepted my limitations and committed to practicing as much as I could, I became more comfortable and capable in all sorts of conditions. I discovered that, even when I was out of my element, I felt equipped to roll with whatever gnarly waves came my way.

It's the same with MS. Your symptoms, like the conditions of the ocean, will be changeable—and some "waves" will seem more manageable than others. In the face of the "gnarliest," I've found that *rolling with it* opens me up to learning new ways of navigating. I may conquer my symptoms, or they may hurl me into the trough—but either way, the experience is an adventure.

I hope this book helps you better surf the waves of your own condition and symptoms, discover some wisdom, and perhaps even gain an appreciation for the adventure along the way.

than humans. After all, animal vocabulary is simpler: *woof* and *meow*, versus an onerous number of syllables in complex combinations!

I also felt connected in new ways to people who had difficulty in speaking—like my former neighbor with Down syndrome whom I'd occasionally see in and around town. My condition changed the nature of my relationships, and whom I communicated with. Now when I saw him in town, we would play patty-cake with our hands, and he would just smile. I didn't need to expect any words from him.

I'm not the same person I was before MS. But I'm thankful that I can pursue my work to understand, and confront, my illness.

This book represents the fruits of my quest in being whole even while my identity, my personality, was eroded. It's not a solution, or a miracle cure, for MS; it is a realistic attempt to understand and manage the illness—and feel well and whole—as much as possible, for as long as possible.

Although I spent a significant portion of my 40s living with debilitating symptoms, I am grateful to have enjoyed moments and days of clarity and to have continued working. Rather than focusing my life on sleep and rest, I adopted the philosophy of creating adequate time for sleep and rest, while pursuing life within my new limitations. With the assistance of dedicated and skilled staff, I launched the *Journal of Restorative Medicine*, the Restorative Medicine Conference, and a medical association that has more than 500 members. I'm not trying to brag by sharing these accomplishments. My

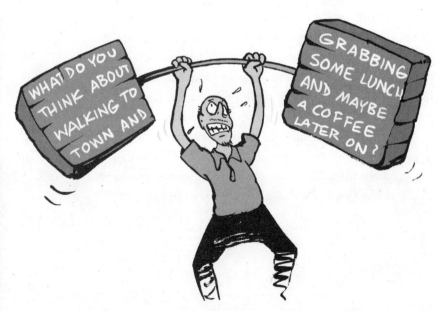

For those with the cognitive brain fog of MS, it's a lot of work to make sense of a pile of words coming from conversations.

message is that despite the difficulties MS can bring, it is completely possible to live a fulfilling life.

I hope that what I've found will be useful as you and your loved ones navigate the difficult course of this challenging disease. And although the advice in this book is specific to multiple sclerosis, it can also serve as a useful guidepost for treating all neurological diseases, especially those with autoimmune implications, such as Parkinson's, Alzheimer's, and others.

MS remains a serious disease without a cure. But researchers are working to deconstruct and solve its mysteries. They haven't yet determined how to fully stop MS in its tracks. But aided by tools, techniques, and insights that have never before been available, researchers are helping patients to slow the progression of their disease.

Today, 10 years after first being diagnosed with MS, I believe I possess a much deeper, and more nuanced, understanding of it. Based on continued advances in the field, on my own research, and personal trial and error, I've grown and refined my naturopathic tool kit. (In fact, as I describe in chapter 7, some of the specific tools in this kit have led to decreased lesions in my brain, as measured by MRI. Some lesions have even disappeared!) And I've learned some promising approaches to manage the disease in a way I hadn't been able to before. Beyond seeing MS "simply" as an autoimmune disease—as I had when first diagnosed—I now grasp the full breadth of its pathophysiological causes. Neurological health conditions like MS involve multiple complex relationships among many systems in the body. Across medical practices, it connects immunology (it's an autoimmune disease), gastroenterology (the microbiome in the human gut impacts neurotransmitters), and endocrinology (the myelin sheath is stimulated by thyroid hormones). Psychology and psychoneuroimmunology are connected, too, because as with all illnesses, the mind has a big influence on how we react to MS.

CHAPTER 2

The Ones Who Leave the Jungle

"The only people who get sick are the ones who leave the jungle." This is what my friend Juan Uyunkar, a Shuar medicine man from the Amazon in Ecuador, told me about his people. He noticed that those who stayed true to their traditional lifestyle in the jungle never suffered from chronic disease. Every day, traditionally they walked to gather bananas. They fished and hunted for their food. But once Shuar people, including Juan himself, moved to the cities, where they were exposed to pollution, stress, and a diet of fast food, they developed a host of chronic diseases that were unheard-of in the rain forest.

To understand why this happened, let's look at the parallels between the human body and an organic farm. Organic farmers seek to provide a *balanced ecosystem* for their crops: using natural methods to build nutrient-rich soil free of chemical fertilizers and pesticides, in the climate and conditions appropriate for the produce they grow. When the balance is right, the crops are healthy and productive, but any disruptions to the ecosystem's delicate equilibrium can lead to disease and, possibly, crop failure.

The same is true for humans. When something in our environment is out of whack, we can, and often do, become sick.

In 1995—while a student at the Canadian College of Naturopathic Medicine —I visited the native community in the Mohawk Territory. They told me about the explosion of autoimmune disorders among the First Nation communities in the region.

For centuries these peoples had lived off the land: hunting, fishing, and farming while enjoying relative freedom from the "diseases of modernity."

But something had changed in the past few decades. Hypo- and hyperthy-roidism and other chronic disease had become endemic. As I rode in a boat up the St. Lawrence River with some of the locals, they pointed out that these very waters, in which the people fished, were directly downstream from the Reynolds Metals Company and General Motors. Those manufacturing plants were dumping polychlorinated biphenyls (PCBs) and halogenated aromatic compounds—chlorine, bromine, and fluorine—into the rivers, contaminating the fish and surrounding soils. Each of these compounds is directly implicated in the development of autoimmune disease.

The natural resources of the Mohawk communities, and their tradition-ally clean way of living, had literally been poisoned. Through ingesting the toxins dumped by Reynolds and GM, the First Nation tribes in Mohawk Ter-ritory were suffering serious negative effects, in the form of chronic disease. Simply put, they were victims of environmental racism.

The Shuar and the Mohawk are not the only people affected by industrial pollutants and compromised diets. The facts are hard to escape: In the last 50 years alone, the rates of autoimmune diseases such as multiple sclerosis have doubled. *Doubled!* Notably, these increases are occurring in first-world countries where daily exposures to chemicals and other toxins are common; where an over-reliance on antibiotics leads to disturbances in gut microflora; and where stress is simply a fact of life. When the human ecosystem is dis-rupted, the organism risks disease.

Our knowledge of other indigenous cultures further supports this theory. For example, studies of Bolivia's Tsimane peoples reveal that they have the cleanest arteries of any culture on Earth, with no evidence of cardiovascular disease. They also seem to experience cognitive *increases*, rather than the expected declines, when the ApoE4 gene (which is associated with Alzhei-mer's disease) is present. Researchers believe that the unique composition of the Tsimanes' gut flora influences gene expression in a beneficial way.

Toxins, Diet, and Disease

Of course, at the time that I was discovering these connections among toxins, diet, and disease, I had no idea how personally relevant they would become. Once I began learning more about MS, however, and the internal and external factors that contribute to it, I understood how addressing these factors in a holistic way could help my body return to its desired uncorrupted state—giving me the best chance for staving off progression of the disease.

One of the most important steps in protecting brain health is to minimize exposures to damaging toxins from external sources and to enhance detoxification of the body to deal with any offenders already present in your system. Many chemicals commonly used in household products, in manufacturing, and in agriculture act as endocrine disruptors, meaning they bind to hormone receptor sites and have deleterious effects.

One example is perfluorooctanoate (PFOA), a chemical used to make nonstick kitchenware, as well as stain- and water-resistant fabric and carpets (think Teflon and Gore-Tex). Flame retardants, polybrominated diphenyl ethers (PBDEs), bisphenol A (BPA), and phthalates in plastics, atrazine in .herbicides, organophosphates in pesticides, mercury in certain types of fish (as well as dental fillings, some vaccines, and fluorescent lightbulbs), and others are also considered endocrine disruptors. These chemicals also have contaminated our water supply and the soil in which our food is grown. One of the many problems with these chemicals is that they are very stable and break down slowly. Therefore they remain in the environment, our food supply, and our body for a very long time.[1] It is impossible to find a place on this planet that is devoid of these toxins.

Preliminary research suggests multiple ways that these toxins damage the brain, such as directly damaging neurons, attaching to hormone receptor sites and altering their actions, disrupting neurotransmitter production, and more. Worse, scientists speculate that toxins may alter genes in a way that passes down the damage to future generations. Much more research is needed to accurately pinpoint the extent to which environmental toxins contribute to MS, Alzheimer's, and other health problems, and how to best resolve these problems.[2]

Centuries of Mystery

While the origins and first cases of the disease now known as multiple sclerosis have been lost to time, the earliest recorded descriptions date back to the Middle Ages. It wasn't until the early 1800s, however, that Scottish physician and professor of pathology Robert Carswell first discovered the spinal cord plaques (lesions) that characterize the condition—although he didn't know what the plaques were, or what effects they exerted on the patients who had them.[3] (He observed the plaques during postmortem examinations, which precluded any direct questioning.)

Eventually, Jean-Martin Charcot figured it out. Known today as the Father of Neurology, Dr. Charcot was a French physician and professor whose many students at the University of Paris included a young Sigmund Freud. For many years, as his predecessors had, Charcot struggled to effectively manage patients suffering from a mystery illness with a baffling, and varied, array of symptoms. In 1868, when one of these patients died, her autopsy told the story: distinctive lesions on her brain that Charcot correctly connected to her previously unexplained tremors, slurred speech, and involuntary eye movements. He called these lesions *sclerose en plaques*. With that, the disease finally had a name.

Despite this significant diagnostic discovery, Dr. Charcot never successfully treated a case of MS. He tried many approaches common at the time, including injections of gold and silver, electrical stimulation, and minute dosages of the poison strychnine. All of these treatments are known to stimulate nerves, but none had any significant impact on the MS patients.

It was not until the early 1900s that researchers uncovered the next important piece of the puzzle. In the decades since Charcot had identified multiple sclerosis, practitioners had learned that MS struck women more often than men. This seemed to suggest a genetic component, but the condition was not strictly driven by genetics. In 1916, using microscopy, the pathologist Dr. James Dawson of the University of Edinburgh identified two additional characteristics of the disease: inflammation of the blood vessels and damage to the myelin sheath that insulates and protects nerves in the brain and spinal cord. Still, no one knew what caused the plaques, the inflammation, or the myelin damage. Some blamed viruses, which had recently been discovered by the medical community. Others pointed to environmental toxins.

Almost 20 years later, in 1935, Dr. Thomas Rivers—a bacteriologist working at The Rockefeller Institute for Medical Research—injected laboratory monkeys with rabbit myelin as part of his investigation into multiple sclerosis. His experiment led to a remarkable discovery: The monkeys developed acute central nervous system reactions marked by damage to their own myelin. In the absence of any identifiable infectious agents introduced through the injections, Rivers concluded that the rabbit myelin was to blame. His work proffered both a plausible cause for the disease and an explanation for its devastating effects. In multiple sclerosis, he posited, the immune system misidentifies myelin as an alien invader and mounts an attack. The resulting damage, or demyelination, causes nerves to misfire and, in some cases, cease to function altogether—which leads to ineffective communication between the brain and the rest of the body. Today researchers continue to use Rivers's groundbreaking experimental model—now known as experimental allergic encephalomyelitis (EAE)—in their quest to better understand multiple sclerosis and other demyelinating diseases.

In the decades since, investigators have developed a much better understanding of multiple sclerosis, its mechanisms, and its contributing factors. I'd like to share what I've learned about these topics through my own quest for information. I'll start with a description of symptoms and some contributing factors.

Symptoms of Multiple Sclerosis

As I've explained in chapter 1, multiple sclerosis is a chronic, autoimmune, inflammatory neurological disease of the central nervous system (CNS). In both presentation and etiology, the disease is complex and notoriously difficult to pin down—as my own story so aptly illustrates. Some of its more common symptoms include:

- Numbness or weakness in one or more limbs that typically occurs on one side of the body at a time, or in the legs and trunk*
- Partial or complete loss of vision, usually in one eye at a time, often with pain during eye movement*
- Prolonged double vision*
- Tingling or pain in parts of the body*
- Electric-shock sensations that occur with certain neck movements, especially bending the neck forward (Lhermitte's sign)*
- Tremor, lack of coordination, or unsteady gait*
- Slurred speech*

- Fatigue*
- Dizziness*
- Problems with bowel and bladder function*
- Taste changes*
- Difficulty chewing and/or swallowing*
- Cardiac issues*
- Breathing irregularity*
- Loss of hearing*
- Short-term memory loss*
- Problems with executive functioning such as planning*
- Problems with memory, attention span, and impulse control*
- Problems with information processing*

Because no two patients experience the same symptoms in the same way with the same frequency, intensity, or duration, diagnosing MS can often be more art than science. One patient may present with a single symptom; another with *all* of them. One patient's tremors might be mild; another's, completely debilitating. And so on. Practitioners, then, must rely on their knowledge, experience, and intuition in order to appropriately characterize each case into one of the four main subtypes.[4]

As explained in chapter 1, relapsing-remitting MS (RRMS) is the most common subtype of the disease. It's the form I live with, and it constitutes up to 85 percent of cases. In RRMS symptoms arise and persist for a defined (though individually variable) period of time that can last for days, weeks, or months. (Some symptoms, especially those that continue for more than a year or two, can become permanent.) During periods of remission, when the disease is neither active nor progressing, these symptoms can wane, sometimes for years, before they return. Notably, however, remission doesn't mean that patients escape *every* symptom. For example, I typically in the past experienced an annual MS attack (flare-up) in the spring, which is fairly common for most RRMS patients. (Some studies suggest this might be due to an inverse relationship between the hormone melatonin, which is naturally lower during the

---

* Yep, I've had 'em all.

spring and summer for people living in northern climates, and disease activity. I talk more about this in chapter 7.) During these attacks, I experience more severe cognitive difficulties, motor impairments, and urinary dysfunction than I do in "calmer" phases of the disease—although these symptoms never truly disappear. I also battle other symptoms, including fatigue, paresthesia (a prickling or burning sensation), and issues with peristalsis (the involuntary movement that pushes food, digestive by-products, and microbes through the gut), throughout the year. In secondary progressive MS (SPMS), symptoms steadily worsen over time. Most patients who suffer from RRMS eventually transition to the secondary progressive form of the disease. In my case, I have successfully staved off this progression for more than 20 years. In large part, I attribute this to the strategies I detail in the remainder of this book.

In primary progressive MS (PPMS), which makes up about 10 percent of cases, symptoms arise and persist without remission, and can rapidly progress. And clinically isolated syndrome (CIS) can be tricky. CIS describes an initial episode of neurological symptoms consistent with neuroinflammation or demyelination followed by complete recovery. Patients may experience just one symptom, such as acute aphasia (the inability to speak), that correlates to a single lesion; or a cluster of symptoms caused by more than one lesion. Many individuals who experience CIS eventually develop full-blown disease, though some don't. Continued research and improvements to MRI technology will help with more precise diagnosis.

Because the symptoms of multiple sclerosis are so variable and can quickly become debilitating, it is important to seek immediate medical advice and care should any of them occur. It's also important to understand that although the symptoms of MS are well documented, their variable nature often results in misdiagnoses, such as in my case. For this reason, practitioners must look beyond a patient's clinical presentation in order to accurately diagnose the disease.

Ordinarily, a physician who suspects MS will order an MRI of the patient's brain and spinal cord. This close-up look at the central nervous system is truly the "gold standard" for diagnosis, as it reveals the characteristic demyelinated lesions, or plaques, that give multiple sclerosis its name. In the absence of such plaques, which appear as white areas on an MRI, practitioners can confidently rule out the condition.

Multiple Sclerosis Risk Factors

Age. MS can occur at any age, but most commonly affects people between the ages of 15 and 60.

Sex. Women are four times as likely as men to develop MS.

Ethnic background. White people, particularly those of Northern European descent, are at higher risk for MS. It was thought that people of Asian, African, and Native American descent had a lower risk profile than Caucasians of Northern European ancestry. However, it is unclear whether this is because research has not focused as much on these populations until recently. It is known that MS symptoms and relapse rates can be more severe in African Americans.

Family history. If one of your parents or siblings has, or had, MS, you are at higher risk of developing the disease.

Certain autoimmune diseases. You have a slightly higher risk of developing MS if you already have thyroid disease, type 1 diabetes, or inflammatory bowel disease.

Certain infections. While none has been definitively identified as causative, several viruses have been *linked* to MS—including Epstein-Barr, which is responsible for infectious mononucleosis. Certain gastrointestinal parasites, such as *Clostridium* bacteria, may also play a role. Perhaps having an unhealthy microbiome could even be a trigger.

Climate. MS is far more common in countries with temperate climates, including Canada, the northern United States, New Zealand, southeastern Australia, and Europe.

Smoking. Smokers who experience initial symptoms suggestive of MS are more likely than nonsmokers to develop additional symptoms consistent with relapsing-remitting MS (RRMS).

Today, building on Dr. Rivers's 1935 discovery of *how* these plaques form, researchers have begun to better understand *why* they form. The reasons involve a critical physiological structure known as the blood-brain barrier (BBB): a semipermeable layer of cells that restricts the passage of harmful substances, such as bacteria and neurotoxins, from the bloodstream into the brain and central nervous system. MS is characterized by transient or chronic disruption of the BBB. It's not known whether this "leakiness" is a factor in the *cause* of MS or whether it's a *consequence* of having the disease. Simply put, a leaky BBB is tied in closely with MS. We do know that in multiple sclerosis, *leukocytes* (white blood cells) cross the BBB and infiltrate the myelin sheath. Some studies also suggest that specialized cells in the CNS called *microglial cells*—which function to clean up debris, among other things—try to halt the damage created by leukocyte infiltration. However, in so doing, the microglial cells actually cause the demyelination that characterizes MS— the body *attacks itself.* I discuss this in more detail in chapter 3.

Cognitive Effects of Multiple Sclerosis

In medicine, an aphorism credited to medical researcher Dr. Theodore Woodward applies: "When you hear hoofbeats, think horses, not zebras." When I consulted my family doctor and others about the first signs that something was going drastically wrong with my health, those physicians didn't recognize the bold black-and-white stripes of multiple sclerosis. That's probably because I was an otherwise young, healthy man, and it was much more likely that my cognitive symptoms such as short-term memory loss and inability to pay attention were due to a common, more benign cause like food poisoning or a urinary tract infection: a "horse," in other words.

And yet, according to the National Multiple Sclerosis Society, as many as half of the estimated one million patients living with the disease in the United States experience problems with cognition: those advanced brain functions including "the ability to learn and remember information, organize, plan and problem-solve, focus, maintain and shift attention, understand and use language, accurately perceive the environment, and perform calculations."[5] Further, according to the society, problems with cognition may be the *first* symptom of multiple sclerosis most people experience. That was true in my case. Still, many health care providers who do not specialize in treating the disease believe that neuropsychological effects are rare. Among the hundreds of thousands of people who are affected, however, such disturbances present a very real, very stressful, and often heartbreaking daily challenge for them and their caregivers.

Generally speaking, these cognitive impairments bear little relation to other manifestations of the MS: Someone with excellent mobility can suffer serious cognitive issues, while a patient who is significantly disabled physically can remain cognitively unaffected. And it's important to note that comorbidities—factors that exist simultaneously with the multiple sclerosis disease process—can impact cognitive function, too. Fatigue, stress, nutritional deficiencies, hormone imbalances, insomnia, and even things like normal aging can exacerbate symptoms.

Many patients also struggle with psychological effects that are due both to the disease itself (damaged neurons and neurotransmitters), and to the challenges of living with it every day. In rare cases patients can experience symptoms that are so severe, they lose their sense of control. Left unaddressed, these symptoms can lead to social isolation, depression, substance abuse, and other self-destructive behaviors. In fact, studies have shown that the suicide rate among multiple sclerosis patients is almost double that of the general population.[6] This is why it's so important to understand, recognize, and treat the cognitive manifestations of the disease early.

That's the bad news. The good news—as I have learned through my own personal experiences and extensive research—is that there are effective ways not only to manage, but also to reduce, the impacts of these symptoms. Pharmaceuticals, botanical medicines, nootropics, and lifestyle activities such as memory games, organizational aids, and reminders are all great ways to manage cognitive symptoms. Nootropics, also known as smart drugs, are supplements and drugs that improve memory, executive functions, and motivation.

Before we delve into how to apply these tools, let's discuss some of the most common cognitive impacts of multiple sclerosis and how to recognize them. (I discuss the strategies for managing these impacts separately, later in the chapter.) Researchers are still working to identify the full complement of cognitive processes and functions that might be affected in those with multiple sclerosis, but several consistently surface among patients worldwide. According to the National Multiple Sclerosis Society, the most common of these are memory disturbances, attention deficits, and delays in information processing, visual-spatial abilities, and verbal fluency.

Memory Disturbances

Memory disturbance is the cognitive effect that MS patients most frequently report experiencing. As with Alzheimer's, multiple sclerosis tends to affect a patient's ability to remember experiences in the recent, rather than distant, past. (It's important to note that the disease pathways are different, however; for many MS patients, issues with cognition progress slowly and may wax and wane over time.) In some MS patients, memory itself isn't actually the problem; instead, they experience attention deficits and problems processing information, which can make it difficult both to access important details and to adequately learn recently presented ones, such as a new acquaintance's name.

I recall one evening when I wrote a rather incoherent note to my family because I was experiencing cognitive issues, and I wanted to let them know I loved them just in case I wouldn't remember who they were the following day. The imagery of a storm was my poetic way of describing that something was changing fast in my body. What was happening in my thoughts would later be confirmed in an MRI indicating a small new lesion in my frontal brain, where processing information and memory would be impacted. The following week I experienced a few seconds' delay before I could recognize my three-year-old son. There are many adventures in MS. As I mentioned before, one never knows what our future array of symptoms might be. For me, this inability to recognize my son—thankfully a fleeting problem—was

Wind is coming, , coming and storm will was here, I And hope in sunrise that' I may Know Know the the ppeople I love, hope my my family will I know

In this note I wrote the night before one of my early attacks, it's clear to see that my thinking is garbled. At the time I wasn't really familiar with all the symptoms of MS. I was feeling confused, and I couldn't sequence time correctly.

the symptom that made me the saddest. It left me even more focused on trying to find the holy grail and looking for the cure.

Experiences like these were among the first markers of my own disease, as evidenced by my visit to Burlington, Vermont—a place I know well—and becoming utterly lost.

I now understand, thanks to my journey with this disease, that I will always face occasional episodes of memory loss. But I'm much better equipped to weather their challenges. Many times, I can even predict when they might occur.

Attention Deficits

After I learned that I had multiple sclerosis, certain aspects of my life made a lot more sense to me: like the way I couldn't absorb the meaning of things Sarika would say to me if I was doing something else—even something as simple as getting dressed. I just thought I was a poor multitasker; as it turns out, MS had compromised my ability to maintain adequate focus when more than one person or task competed for my attention.

Everyone, whether living with MS or not, has experienced this phenomenon at one time or another. (We all know a person who "can't walk and chew gum" at the same time. And maybe it's us!) For MS patients, though, the challenges of divided attention are much more acute and tend to affect situations that most other people could easily manage, like watching television while washing the dishes. Or following a conversation at the dinner table while also eating one's meal. But keep in mind that certain MS patients have trouble learning new things. Because these patients process information much more slowly than others, they require a lot more time to absorb and retain what they learn. When they don't have the benefit of that time—when they can't fully focus on a single task or conversation—they struggle. And the feeling of constant distraction can be exceptionally frustrating, for both patients and their loved ones.

Delays in Information Processing

In Europe the norm in many countries is to drive on the left-hand side of the road rather than the right. You've probably heard stories of American travelers who, unaccustomed to the "new" rules of the road, pull out of the car rental lot and immediately start driving in the wrong lane. Maybe you've even done it yourself! It probably happens hundreds of times a day across the Continent. Most times, drivers immediately notice signs of their mistake and act quickly to correct it. That's because, unlike MS patients like me, they can rapidly absorb, make sense of, and react to information—such as the movement of other cars, a streetlight oriented away from the lane they're traveling in, or a passenger yelling "wrong side!" from the next seat.

Some MS patients literally have trouble keeping up. When the disease impacts this area of cognition, it takes much longer to think things through and respond: It's like we're stuck in the slow lane while everyone else is speeding by. It's not that we *can't* understand the situation; we just require extra time and space to figure it out. In turn, this can affect our ability to analyze and respond to issues, weigh the pros and cons of even simple decisions, solve both abstract and concrete problems, and plan a course of action. Without understanding from family and friends, our actions might be interpreted as offensive. For example, while walking through town, a friend and I made a plan to eat at a restaurant for lunch. While confirming the details, I heard a car pass by, which distracted me, and I wasn't able to remember and process the commitment to meet for lunch an hour later. So I never showed up at the restaurant. Years later, my friend told me he felt like I "blew him off" and wasn't interested in being friends anymore. Like attention deficits, these challenges are also closely related to memory, attention, and learning. But a few simple strategies can reduce their impact.

In working to manage this cognitive slowdown, I have learned that one of the best things I can do is to conserve my energy so that it's available when I need to make important decisions—and to take my time in doing so. Another successful strategy I use is to limit my involvement in situations and relationships that aren't positive, which helps prevent mental fatigue.

Visual-Spatial Abilities

I vividly recall a couple of examples of problems with my visual-spatial abilities that occurred before I'd been diagnosed with MS. One day my mother-in-law offered me tea—and I saw four hands, with four cups,

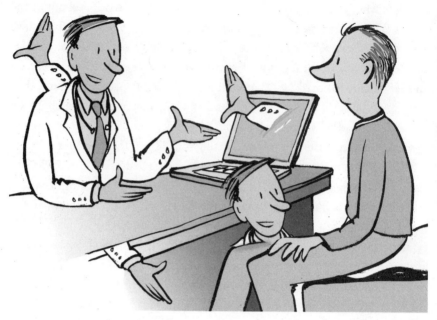

The weird tricks that MS plays, like this otherworldly scene I once experienced while visiting an emergency room, make for a funny story, but in real time they are thoroughly disorienting. As it turned out, I had a lesion in the area of my brain that controls *visuospatial* functions—the ability to see and perceive a scene accurately and to draw or assemble objects.

extending toward me, as if she were an Indian goddess. Later the same day, in the emergency room, I felt like I'd been dropped onto the set of a psychedelic film from the 1970s: the doctor's disembodied head appeared perched on my knee; and one of his hands sprouted from his shoulder while the other poked out from his computer monitor. *What is wrong with me? I wondered. Is this forever?*

People who have normal visuospatial function likely take it for granted. But it's absolutely crucial for everyday tasks such as walking across a room without smashing into a piece of furniture, loading a dishwasher, putting furniture together, or operating a car. Although I still occasionally suffer episodes of disordered vision that can last as long as six months, it happens much less frequently than it used to, and lasts a shorter amount of time, thanks to the treatments I've used.

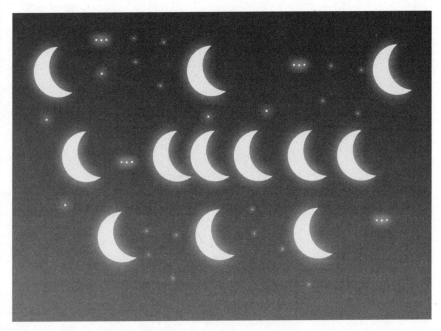

I've also had the unusual experience of seeing as many as 15 moons shining in the night sky. This is due to failure of the nerve signals in my eyes to align with one another. It's a beautiful sight, but this kind of disordered vision makes it impossible to drive safely.

Verbal Fluency

Have you ever wanted to use a specific word but just couldn't "spit it out"? Most of us have experienced temporary language difficulties like this. Patients with MS, however, deal with fluency issues pretty frequently—and they're likely related to problems with memory and information processing.

Others, myself included, have also struggled with short moments of *aphasia* —the inability to speak, understand others, and even read or write.

Before I was diagnosed—but after I'd already begun experiencing many other cognitive symptoms of MS—I experienced episodes in which a simple sentence from a loved one sounded like a jumbled heap of nonsense. Rearranging their words into a coherent sequence was exhausting—or even impossible. It worked the other way around, too. It sometimes took an interminable amount of time for me to figure out which words to use,

---

I have Aphasia

Aphasia affects my ability to SPEAK and can also affect reading, writing, and understanding. *My intellect is not affected*—only language!

Please take time to communicate with me:

- Speak SLOWLY and CLEARLY   · Ask YES/NO questions
- Use SHORT sentences   · Shouting doesn't help
- Give me TIME to respond   · Keep it SIMPLE

Thank you for your patience and understanding!

When my first speech therapist gave me this card, I threw it away, because it felt disempowering and I believed I wouldn't need it.

and in what order. It felt as though I were back in college physics, facing a complicated equation I had no idea how to solve. The difficulty was so great that at times I didn't even want to bother trying to talk.

As you might imagine, aphasia can easily snowball into social isolation, which can lead to depression. Even though my case was very mild, I withdrew not just from group situations, but also from interactions with certain friends. Hanging out with guy friends can involve a lot of bantering and joking around. It took me as long as five minutes to understand one of my friend's jokes and then respond, but by then another set of jokes was already starting. It did make me feel isolated, so I stopped getting together with them. The wife of one of my best friends had a good friend with MS who would just hold up her hand and say "Stop!" to indicate that she needed some time to process the conversation before she could continue talking. This is helpful, and having friends and family who recognize that this kind of signal can be helpful is very supportive.

A speech therapist gave me an aphasia communication card after I experienced an episode in which I wasn't able to talk for 15 minutes. I've shown the card to one friend, who thought it was really funny. But people on the outside, who don't see me often, would never believe I could have problems like those described on the card, because 99 percent of the time I don't. And during those limited times I feel it's hard to speak clearly, I don't leave the house. I don't think my friend's laughter was mean-spirited, it was just a reaction to an uncomfortable situation of listening to a friend admit to a problem, especially a problem that is almost never visible to others.

I've also undergone intensive speech therapy, in my case over a period of years. While duration times vary, this is another specific strategy I highly recommend. Speech therapists can help with much more than just verbal fluency. I also had problems with the muscles that control speech; weakness in mine made it hard to speak loudly enough to be heard, which made it difficult to socialize. I also had laryngospasms, or sudden spasms in my vocal cords, and dysfunctional synchronizing between both bilateral vocal cords. This diagnosis was based on yet another tube inserted in my body (the first being a urinary catheter due to urinary retention). The second tube contained a camera, which was inserted through my nose into my throat. It revealed that my speaking muscles weren't functioning in symmetry. The right side would work, while the left side didn't. To treat these conditions, my speech therapist gave me exercises to rebuild my vocal cord muscles. To maintain the progress I worked so hard to achieve, I continue them to this day, practicing for 15 minutes most mornings. When I skip them—I'm human!—my symptoms do unfortunately recur. When those muscles are weak, it also causes issues with swallowing.

People who were unaware of my diagnosis when they first met me report they would never have known I had MS by simply talking with me, and that's a welcome reward for all of the hard work and effort I have devoted to speech therapy.

Managing Cognitive Symptoms

Current research indicates that of those MS patients who are affected by cognitive changes, only about 5 to 10 percent suffer moderate to severe impairment—which sounds like good news. However, it's difficult to apply these definitions consistently from one patient to another. A person's age, what they do for a living, where they live and with whom, and even their general outlook on life can all be determining factors in how particular symptoms impact their lives, and how they cope. Even mild visuospatial disturbances could end a young concert pianist's career, for example.

My Personal Prescription for Managing Cognitive Symptoms

Here's a summary of foods, herbs, supplements, therapies, and life-style adjustments that can help to reduce the impact of the cognitive symptoms that MS patients may experience. There's more information about all of these recommendations throughout this book. Whenever possible, choose whole organic foods.

Do eat:

- A variety of fruits and berries, including avocados, citrus, kiwi, blueberries, raspberries, and strawberries
- Nuts and seeds, including flaxseeds and walnuts
- Vegetables, including broccoli, butternut squash, and dark leafy greens
- Salmon and other fish
- Healthy oils, including coconut oil and olive oil
- Dark chocolate
- Red wine
- Eggs

Don't eat:

- Junk food or processed foods

Choose these herbs and supplements:

- Lion's mane mushroom (not mycelium)
- *Bacopa monnieri*
- *Cordyceps sinensis*
- Rosmarinic acid
- Glutathione
- T3 thyroid hormones
- Modafinil

- Piracetam
- Pharmaceuticals that reduce MS progression

Take part in:
- Your favorite exercise
- Speech therapy
- Occupational therapy

Practice:
- Conserving energy
- Planning chores in advance
- Using lists and labels
- Meditation

At the time I was diagnosed, I was an endocrinology instructor at a university, and my schedule was demanding. I continued to teach until I founded the Association for the Advancement of Restorative Medicine and assumed its directorship, and still haven't applied for the disability benefits I refused when I was first diagnosed. My point here is that it doesn't really matter where cognitive impacts fall on the spectrum of mild to severe, because they're all relative. I am fortunate to have been able to continue my work, but that doesn't mean my symptoms haven't been severe at times.

Piracetam is a nootropic or smart drug, commonly used to promote mental performance. It is available under various brand names, including Nootropil and Lucetam. Most of the research on piracetam is dated, but it has been shown to provide benefits that could be helpful for people with MS. It seems to protect against myoclonic seizures, which are characterized by sudden, painful muscle spasms or involuntary movements, both of which can occur with MS.[7] Studies also show that piracetam improves aspects of mental performance, such as memory, reaction time, and ability to focus in people with Alzheimer's disease and other forms of cognitive impairment.[8]

Piracetam is generally considered low risk. Long-term studies have shown that doses up to 24 grams a day are well tolerated. It may interact with other medications, however, so please consult with your health care provider before trying it.

I have tried taking many herbs and supplements recommended for cognitive enhancement. Modafinil, which is a dopamine agonist/stimulant, initially worked well for me but then began to cause heart palpitations. Today I use Ocrevus, and I'm happy to say it has made a huge difference in my quality of life in terms of cognitive function, such as planning and memory function. It isn't a perfect solution, and I still struggle with cognitive difficulties from time to time. However, I've learned to stay relaxed and be tolerant of these symptoms when they occur.

CHAPTER 3

A Loss of Balance

When I was a practicing physician, one of my first patients was an autistic woman who could not talk. The patient foamed at the mouth with white sputum. She spat on everyone she saw—I was told to wear a rain jacket when I met with her. As it turned out, that was good advice. As part of my diagnostic workup of this patient, I did a urine test, which revealed large amounts of yeast breakdown products and the presence of two heavy metals: cadmium and lead.

The patient's caretaker told me that she had been institutionalized as a child and had often been strapped in a chair (in the days when that was still legal). During those times, she ate chips of blue paint from the walls—paint that contained those two toxic substances.

In an effort to help the patient, I prescribed dimercaptosuccinic acid (DMSA), which helps remove heavy metals from the body. I also gave her antifungals to reduce the overabundance of yeast and put her on an antifungal diet. By killing the yeast in the gut and removing the heavy metals, this treatment improved her condition considerably. She no longer foamed at the mouth, and she was able to sit next to people without hitting and spitting. A change in her gut flora and a reduction in toxic metal had improved the neurological symptoms of autism and made her more personable. She improved so much that the Connecticut Department of Social Services wrote me a letter saying that due to her remarkable changes, they would pay the cost of anything I prescribed, even organically grown food.

The dramatic effects of treating this patient's yeast imbalance in the gut, and her toxic load of cadmium and lead, clearly demonstrated to me that neurology is a fusion of complex interactions between gastroenterology and toxicology.

The Microbiome and Gut Health

What is a microbiome? In a general sense, it is a mutually beneficial biological community comprising bacteria, viruses, fungi, and other specialized microorganisms that—together with their host—work to create and maintain a fully healthy environment. Almost every ecosystem, whether on land, sea, or air, has its own microbiome that has evolved over time to support that ecosystem's life. Specific microbiomes in the forest, for example, collaborate to break down, digest, and recycle organic matter into essential nutrients that foster tree growth. Without this process, the forest could neither survive nor thrive.

Human beings also have a microbiome: what I like to imagine as a giant party in the gut. More than one hundred trillion "guests" (microorganisms) dance in tune with their respective hosts (us). Those microbes "sweat out" metabolites that ultimately regulate and support our every physiological process: our circulation, digestion, metabolism, neurologic function, and immune system, among others. These are truly guests we love to have! In fact, according to a team of researchers out of Stanford University and the University of California–San Francisco, it is "clear that our microbiota [a term often used interchangeably with *microbiome*] is more like an organ than an accessory: These microbes are not just key contributors to human health but a *fundamental component of human physiology*" (emphasis mine).[1] Like those trees in the forest, we literally depend upon our microbiome to survive and thrive.

The Microbiome Census

As many as 40,000 microbial species reside within the human gut—the proportional populations of which depend on nutrition, environmental sterility, antibiotic use, and the presence of disease.

And more than 100 *trillion* individual bacteria, fungi, viruses, and archaea (single-celled organisms without a nucleus) live there, too.

Our microbiome can influence immune system cells in various ways. In research published in the journal *Gut Microbes*, investigators demonstrate that the human microbiome plays a crucial role in the production of interleukin-17 (IL-17)—a key player in immune system function and an essential weapon against certain invasive bacteria and fungi.[2] Research further suggests that imbalances in the gut can lead to imbalances in the immune system. And researchers have also discovered that "specific intestinal microbial species . . . are sufficient to promote disease in the CNS."[3]

The science behind this is rather complex, but it boils down to the fact that the microbiome regulates both anti- and pro-inflammatory responses in the gut and central nervous system. Further, the researchers note, "alterations in the community composition of the microbiota, known as dysbiosis, may be a critical factor in numerous immune-mediated diseases." This means that when the microbiome suffers imbalances, the T cells that help direct the immune response end up misidentifying healthy tissues as a threat. This knocks the immune system out of homeostasis and often triggers autoimmune disease.

Microbiome Variations

Animals depend on microbiomes for healthy functioning, too.

Cattle, for example, depend on the bacteria and protozoans in their guts to digest cellulose—which makes up much of their diet—into short-chain fatty acids and other nutrients.

And leaf-cutter ants require an external microbiome to feed themselves. After excising pieces out of leaves, the ants store the cut pieces in layers much like a compost pile, which encourages bacteria to grow and digest the leaves. As a by-product of this process, fungi that serve as the ants' primary food source flourish, while competing fungi are inhibited by antibiotic-producing microbes. The common thread within these complex ecosystems is the ability to maintain balance through self-regulation.

Although research into this fascinating evolutionary miracle has only recently exploded, our understanding of the gut and its influence on human health and well-being dates back thousands of years. In fact, almost every ancient healing tradition points to the idea that "death begins in the colon."

The Ayurvedic sages of India, for example, speak of *ama*—an accumulation of toxic residue that disrupts the metabolic fire, or *agni*. In order to restore agni, practitioners prescribe one of a variety of cleansing protocols to draw these toxins out of the body's tissues and into the digestive tract for elimination. Similarly, the Shuar healers of the Ecuadorian Amazon follow one of many indigenous healing traditions that ascribe poor health and immune system dysfunction to impure blood. In order to purge this garbage, patients participate in a ceremony during which they consume a particular mixture of herbs and tea called *natem*, and nothing else, for three days. Traditionally speaking, "cleaning the gut" has always been the first critical step toward restoring optimal health. Cleaning the gut is also one way of removing impurities from the blood—what many healing traditions regard as a major cause of immune system dysfunction.

Today modern science has built upon this ancient knowledge. Researchers can now explain some of the precise mechanisms by which a healthy microbiome promotes a healthy human organism—as well as how an unhealthy microbiome, called *dysbiosis*, contributes to a wealth of disorders, including multiple sclerosis. Such "cutting edge" research is truly "old edge" with a new interpretation.

We now know, for example, that the concept of impure blood is a sound one: Research has proven that fully one-third of the molecules in our bloodstream comprise the breakdown products of our own gut microflora. When we suffer from dysbiosis, we literally become "full of garbage": Endotoxins (natural by-products secreted by specific types of bacteria) from our digestive system leak into our bloodstream, where they can trigger a systemic inflammatory response. And the results can be devastating: autoimmune disease, neurological conditions, diabetes and other metabolic disorders, heart disease, and even some cancers. In fact, recent research published in *ASN Neuro* (the American Society for Neurochemistry's journal) links the development of multiple sclerosis to poor dietary habits that increase inflammation. Consuming too many calories, sugar-sweetened drinks, fried foods, and not enough fiber—as well as not getting enough exercise—can exert negative effects on the microbiome.[4]

The Microbiome and Health

It's not surprising that the microbial balance in our gut, in both the numbers of species and the numbers of individual microbes of each species, can dramatically impact our health, given that the microbiome:

- Plays a crucial role in immune system development.
- Assists in metabolic functions such as salvaging dietary sugars, producing short-chain fatty acids, synthesizing vitamins, and metabolizing drugs.
- Produces neurotransmitters, including epinephrine and norepinephrine, both of which are associated with the fight-or-flight response, and dopamine, a mood regulator. (In fact, the microbiome manufactures fully 50 percent of the dopamine supply for the human body.) These same nutrients also feed the gut microbiota that produce the neurotransmitters serotonin and acetylcholine as well as other metabolites that are so important to our health.
- Produces γ-aminobutyric acid (GABA), the central nervous system's chief inhibitory transmitter, known for its calming effects.
- Exerts significant influence on mood and emotions via its role in manufacturing neurotransmitters.

The Institute for Immunity, Transplantation and Infection at the Stanford University School of Medicine includes an academic department devoted to studying the microbiome and its impacts on chronic diseases, including autoimmune disease.

The good news is that you can prevent dysbiosis with commonsense, easy-to-follow strategies that I will outline later in this chapter. In doing so, you can greatly ameliorate the symptoms of MS, and—as I will illustrate through my own personal experience—even potentially alter its progression. But first, let's explore some of the mysteries of the gut. What does a healthy gut look like? How does a healthy gut function? And what causes a healthy gut to deteriorate into dysbiosis and disease?

In its optimal functioning state, the human digestive tract is a remarkable machine—one that absorbs food, water, and other substances, and metabolizes them into nutrients that fuel a variety of physiological processes. These same nutrients also feed the gut microbiota that produce serotonin, acetylcholine, and other metabolites that are so important to our health. (You can read more about these neurotransmitters in the relevant section a little later in this chapter.)

A healthy gut is also critical to a healthy immune system: By destroying pathogens, and excreting them as waste, the microbiota prevent them from escaping into the bloodstream where they can do damage. The gut also "educates" the immune system by training T cells to destroy harmful microorganisms, and to tolerate the beneficial ones that make up the microbiome.

In order to protect itself and the body from attack, the gut employs the intestinal mucosal barrier, commonly known as the intestinal barrier. Comprising a combination of mucosal layers, epithelial tissue, and microbiota, the intestinal barrier is a selectively permeable system of physical and biochemical elements that prevent pathogens and toxins from passing through, and allow the absorption of nutrients, vitamins, and minerals. These actions are supported by a number of biochemical elements, including gastric acid and bile, and antimicrobial peptides.

Healthy functioning of the intestinal barrier depends on a balanced microbiome. As we'll see a little later, however, a number of factors can throw our microbiome out of whack . . . and create the conditions that are ripe for dysbiosis.

The Gut-Brain Axis

The human microbiome exerts tremendous influence on our neurological and immune system health—and the key to understanding this phenomenon lies in a structure known as the gut-brain axis (GBA). I'd like to touch on it briefly here, although we'll return to this concept often throughout the rest of this book.

The GBA is a highly complex, bidirectional neurochemical communication highway that transmits signals between the brain and digestive tract. The pathways by which those signals travel include the central nervous system (CNS), which comprises the brain and spinal cord; the enteric nervous system (ENS), a neural network that can independently operate within the gut; the autonomic nervous system (ANS), which controls the functioning of our internal organs; the neuroendocrine system, which works to maintain the body's homeostasis via the hypothalamus, located near the pituitary gland in the brain; and the neuroimmune system, which protects the brain from pathogens. Communications that occur along the GBA regulate a variety of crucial processes, including peristalsis (the involuntary movement that pushes food, digestive by-products, and microbes through the gut) and the creation and delivery of stress-regulating hormones.

Every day, scientists more fully understand the interplay between the GBA and certain disease states. In fact, interactions between the gut and the brain can influence mood, personality, the experience of pain, and even some higher cognitive functions.

Here's a quick story to help illustrate what I know can seem a complicated concept to grasp (physicians reading along may be familiar with it):

Patients suffering from end-stage liver disease can experience something called *hepatic encephalopathy* (HE)—a complex syndrome caused by nitrogenous substances, such as ammonia, escaping the gut and traveling to the brain, resulting in altered consciousness, the inability to communicate, and personality changes. When these patients receive oral or rectally administered lactulose, they can rapidly recover. This is because the lactulose causes feces and its ammonia by-products to purge out of the gut. This reduces the "leakage" of ammonia from the feces in the gut to the bloodstream. The ammonia effects on neurological function are thereby halted. (You'll read more about leaky gut, and its implications, below.) In addition, certain patients respond well to antibiotics that reduce the numbers of ammonia-producing intestinal bacteria—another indication of the crucial interactions between the gut and the brain.[5]

Just as in the case of HE, better understanding of how the gut and brain communicate with each other can offer valuable clues about a variety of illnesses, including multiple sclerosis. We'll return to this concept a little further down. But first, let's explore some of the factors that contribute to an unhealthy gut.

Antibiotics

Antibiotic overuse on a global scale has led to unintended and highly danger-ous consequences: the rise of so-called superbugs such as methicillin-resistant *Staphylococcus aureus* (MRSA), certain strains of *E. coli* and *Salmonella*, and even the bacteria responsible for bubonic plague.[6] The development and almost universal adoption of broad-spectrum antibiotics—combined with overprescription, patient misuse, and agricultural uses in farm animals and crops—means that these bacteria have evolved to resist traditionally effective treatments. Many of these organisms can now be deadly for children, the elderly, and immunocompromised and other vulnerable individuals. It's safe to say that antibiotics have negatively impacted the global ecosystem.

Thanks to current research, we are also beginning to better understand the deleterious effects of antibiotic use at the individual level. The very term *antibiotic* gives us a clue: *anti*, meaning "against"; and *bio*, meaning "life." When we take such medications—and don't get me wrong, there are some very good and necessary reasons for doing so—they act not only on the bad bacteria we want to kill, but also on the very good bacteria resident in our gut. And this disrupts the delicate balance our microbiome depends upon in order to function effectively.

Have you ever suffered an upset stomach during, or shortly after, a course of antibiotics? This is why: Studies have shown that taking ciprofloxacin (for example) for as few as three to four days negatively affects a person's microbiome, greatly decreasing its diversity and depth.[7] The good news is that, with a little help, the gut can generally recover and return to its optimal state within a week or so. The bad news? In some cases, even a single course of antibiotics can *permanently* change a person's microbiome. In young children—a population among the most highly treated with antibiotics—it appears this risk is even more pronounced, and the resulting disruptions to, and loss of biodiversity in, the microbiome are directly related to metabolic disturbances and abnormal immunologic development.[8]

In many ways today's senior citizens seem to be hardier than their grand-children are: The elderly suffer fewer food and environmental allergies; fewer cases of asthma; and fewer autoimmune disorders than young people do. Why? Because they were never extensively treated with the types and doses

Nature or Nurture?

During the past 30 years, the prevalence of neurological autoimmune diseases such as MS has increased by 3.7 percent worldwide annually. And that number rises dramatically when all autoimmune diseases are considered. For example, the prevalence of autoimmune gastrointestinal diseases such as celiac has more than *tripled* during that time, at a rate of 6.3 percent per year.[9]

These observations suggest that our environment exerts a much stronger influence on disease development than do genetics alone. In fact, our environment can affect whether or not certain genes in our bodies get "turned on." This is why a healthy gut is so important—because it can protect against environmental toxins that can lead to poor health.

of antibiotics or exposed to the many environmental toxins that younger adults and children have been. Of course, older generations faced other serious health risks that we don't even need to consider today—rheumatic fever among them—but generally speaking, they certainly had much healthier and more robust microbiomes.

Poor Diet

Antibiotics aren't the only substances that can throw our microbiomes off balance: what we eat matters, too. Our diet is among the leading influences on microbiome health.[10] To understand why, let's look at how our microbiome functions.

Remember that party in your gut I referred to earlier? Well, imagine if you invited a bunch of guests to your home in the late afternoon—long after lunch and shortly before dinner—and only bothered to set out a few small bowls of snack mix. Chances are good that in short order, your guests would be hungry, possibly cranky, and might even behave badly! The same thing is

My Personal Prescription for a Healthy Microbiome

As you'll read throughout this book, I've used a wide range of therapies to treat my MS—so it's difficult to single out one particular approach that's been the most effective. I *can* say that treating my gut with a combination of herbs, nutrients, and prebiotics has played a critical role. If you're wondering where to start with your own complementary treatment, I recommend it be here.

Do eat:

- A diversity of whole foods. This improves intestinal pH and encourages diversity in the microbiome.
- Fermented foods. The by-products of fermentation can be healing for the gut and may support healthy gut bacteria. Microbes found in fermented foods including yogurt and kefir are also beneficial.
- Probiotics.

Don't eat:

- Sugar, especially high-fructose corn syrup; processed foods; excess carbohydrates (these create pro-inflammatory states).
- Trans fats (partially hydrogenated oils).
- Omega-6 oils without their omega-3 counterparts.

Possibly limit or eliminate:

- Gluten or casein.

Take part in:

- For those who can afford it, fecal microbial transplant. (For more on my experience with this innovative therapy, see chapter 4.)

Speaking of Digestion

Constipation is the most common intestinal complaint for patients living with MS. Fortunately, by increasing the good gut flora and decreasing the bad, constipation can be relieved. Herbs that can help prevent dysbiosis are berberine-containing herbs such as goldenseal, oregano oil, and triphala. For some patients this still will not be enough due to impaired nerve signals to the gastrointestinal tract.

Certain herbal supplements can stimulate peristalsis and provide relief. Herbs such as cascara and castor oil have laxative qualities, which stimulate peristalsis. And 5-hydroxytryptophan (5-HTP)—extracted from the seeds of *Griffonia simplicifolia*, an herb native to Ghana—stimulates serotonin, an important neurotransmitter in the enteric nervous system involved in bowel function.

true of the organisms in your gut: Unless you feed them properly, they will starve and become unable to perform their essential functions. Providing a favorite party food—lots and lots of fiber—will keep the guests in your gut quite happy.

Dietary fiber, in the form of minimally cooked vegetables, fruits, nuts, and legumes, provides the fuel your microbiome needs to keep you healthy. During digestion, your gut bacteria extract calories from the foods you eat, synthesize essential vitamins and nutrients, and produce short-chain fatty acids (SCFAs) that are crucial for nourishing the gut barrier, improving immune system function, and fighting inflammation. And studies have shown a direct correlation between high dietary fiber intake and the number of beneficial bacteria in the gut. The same is true for foods that contain polyphenols (a family of antioxidants); in addition to fruits and vegetables, these include dark chocolate, red wine, tea, and coffee.

Unfortunately, our typical American diet—one high in carbohydrates, sugars, and processed foods—has been shown to *decrease* the biodiversity in our gut. It also deprives the microbiome of its fuel. As a consequence, many gut microbes actually begin feeding on the intestinal lining, which increases its permeability and creates a situation called *leaky gut*.

Here's how that happens. The small intestine contains thousands of *tight junctions*, which are microscopic connections that bind the cells of the intestinal lining together. In a healthy gut, these junctions allow only the nutrients the body needs to pass through and into the bloodstream. Other intestinal matter and digestates, such as harmful microbes and endotoxins (natural by-products secreted by specific types of bacteria), remain within the gut and ultimately safely exit the body during elimination.

A molecule called *zonulin* is responsible for regulating the tight junctions of the intestinal barrier. Serving as a physiological gatekeeper, it allows the passage of good molecules, such as nutrients, from the gut into the bloodstream, where they can be absorbed. However, when damaging factors deregulate this so-called zonulin pathway, normally unacceptable molecules can slip through—where they can potentially cause an unwelcome immune response in genetically susceptible individuals.[11] This places MS patients at higher risk for leaky gut and immune reactions.

Interestingly, MS patients are known to have higher serum levels of zonulin as a response to this protein leaking out from a leaky GI tract.

Considered together with additional evidence linking imbalances in the gut to memory and cognitive impairments, this research holds fascinating promise for better understanding and treating many neurological diseases—including multiple sclerosis.

Research has shown that fully one-third of the molecules in our bloodstream comprise the breakdown products of our own gut microflora. The presence of endotoxins in the blood can trigger a systemic inflammatory response from the body's defense mechanisms. And the results can be devastating: autoimmune disease, neurological conditions, diabetes and other metabolic disorders, heart disease, and even some cancers. In fact, recent research published by the American Society for Neurochemistry links the development of multiple sclerosis to poor dietary habits that increase inflammation. Consuming too many calories, sugar-sweetened drinks, fried foods, and not enough fiber—as well as not getting enough exercise—can exert negative effects on the microbiome.[12]

This syndrome of leaky gut is practically a guarantee that the body's immune system will shift into overdrive. The resulting chronic and systemic

---

Common Zonulin Disrupters

- Flavor enhancers
- Food additives such as the ones that make Gummy Bears opaque, doughnut coatings shiny, and some types of white bread "fluffy"
- Dysbiosis

---

inflammation can then damage the blood-brain barrier, as described later in this chapter.

Chronic Stress

Can you remember a time when you were so nervous you felt sick to your stomach? Maybe it was just before a big school test, or during a first date or an athletic competition, or while speaking in front of a crowd. There's a very good reason why stress can have this effect on us: Our brains and our guts are directly connected via a major nerve. It's called the vagus nerve—the tenth cranial nerve that runs from the base of your brain down into your abdomen —and it constantly carries messages back and forth between the two. Scientists are investigating—and beginning much better to understand—precisely how the human stress response can negatively affect our microbiome.

The Hungarian endocrinologist Hans Selye was perhaps the first to observe that stress—either physical or psychological, or both—is the cause for many major illnesses. His now widely accepted theory of general adaptation syndrome (GAS) comprises a three-part response: alarm (the classic fight-or-flight phase), in which hormones such as cortisol and adrenaline flood the bloodstream in preparation for confronting the stressor; resistance, during which the body either returns to normal (if the stressor is resolved) or remains in a state of high arousal; and, finally, exhaustion (if the stressor persists), when the body's ability to cope is depleted. (Less widely known is the fact that Selye was commissioned to study stress by the tobacco industry, which sought to argue that the deleterious effects of stress on humans far outweighed any negative consequences of tobacco use.)

From an evolutionary standpoint, acute stress—such as that experienced during public speaking—is actually healthy in that it temporarily activates your biological processes to help you perform optimally. Once you successfully complete the task, your body returns to equilibrium: Your hormone levels reset, your blood pressure and respiration drop, and you can mentally and physically relax. Those butterflies in your stomach disappear! Chronic stress, on the other hand—that caused by physical, emotional, or sexual abuse; poverty or hunger; an overly demanding job; anxiety or depression—denies the body the chance to reset. This results in a variety of hormonal imbalances, which Selye connected to the development of high blood pressure, heart disease, rheumatoid arthritis, and even some cancers.

But even before Selye, traditional healers around the world knew that stress caused a variety of ills. They didn't need sophisticated research to prove it, either; the fact that it's a common theme among almost every ancient healing tradition speaks to the fact that the concept is nothing new. Informed

Stress and the Gut

In one study of ICU patients who experienced a stress event, researchers noted rapid proliferation of intestinal microorganisms. Stress, they discovered, had led to a decrease in the patients' secretion of hydrochloric acid—which caused their gastric pH to rise to a level hospitable to the microbes.[13]

Just as a small change in the Earth's temperature can tremendously impact the weather and biodiversity of its inhabitants, so, too, can a small shift in the pH of the GI tract affect the microbiome. Physical or emotional stress can not only create increased risk of infection in a hospital setting but also trigger dysbiosis among the general population.

by their knowledge and contemporary investigations, researchers now know that in times of chronic stress, the acidity in the GI tract increases, which disrupts the biodiversity and function of the gut microflora and damages the intestinal lining—a major double-whammy that fosters increased production of endotoxins that then leak into the bloodstream.

Know this: You can be completely relaxed and stress-free, yet still suffer the effects of MS. As you take steps to mitigate stress as discussed here, be gentle with yourself.

Dysbiosis and Neuroinflammation

Dysbiosis can affect almost every system, every mechanism, and every organ in our bodies: from our digestion to our cognition; from our metabolism to our thyroid function; and from our skin to our eyes. It is truly fascinating science. For the purposes of this book, I focus on the impact of dysbiosis on *neuroinflammation*—an inflammatory response in the brain and spinal cord—and on autoimmune response, especially as they relate to multiple sclerosis. Because, as it turns out, dysbiosis is behind these two other major contributing factors to the disease.

Neuroinflammation is a relatively new term. Just a few decades ago, neuroinflammation was a controversial—and not well understood or accepted—topic in the scientific world. Today it's no longer debated; in fact, it's been embraced as a prominent subject in much of the neurological research. Scientists have come to realize that neuroinflammation plays a critical role in the development of neurodegenerative diseases such as MS, and must be addressed as part of a comprehensive MS treatment plan.

Neuroinflammation is caused by pro-inflammatory *cytokines* (chemical messengers) in the brain and spinal cord, and is associated with depression and dementia, as well as more serious conditions such as neurodegeneration. (*Cytokine* is an overall term used to describe an entire group of these messengers, some of which—as you'll see later in this book—can counteract inflammation. These are called anti-inflammatory cytokines.) Neuroinflammation happens at the intersection of the nervous and immune systems. Microglia, the innate immune cells of the central nervous system, perform immune surveillance and control the immune functions of the CNS. They trigger pro-inflammatory signals that can create neurotoxins that damage the CNS. Chronically overactive microglia can create ongoing inflammation that contributes to pathological changes such as neuron damage, depression, and cognitive dysfunction.[14] In the case of MS, acute inflammation can be a positive response from the demyelination of nerves, while chronic inflammation can cause the symptoms that are part of the disease.

Inflammation does serve a purpose in healing, and it can be beneficial under certain circumstances. In some conditions, such as the presence of a CNS infection, an acute, short-lived inflammatory immune response helps eliminate the pathogenic source of the infection, so healing can begin. In such a situation, the brain and immune system communicate with each other to recruit microglia and activate healing. Here, neuroinflammation is highly beneficial and neuroprotective, rather than destructive. Chronic inflammation, on the other hand, can occur when the CNS immune response stops self-regulating, creating a perpetual cycle that can lead to neurodegeneration.

Neuroinflammation can occur through many inflammatory pathways. The type of immune cells that create the inflammation related to MS, for instance, are different from the type that cause Alzheimer's disease and dementia, although the end result is the same. The technical differences lie in the specific types of immune cells and cytokines that are triggered.

These scientific nuances are mainly a concern to researchers and physicians. The take-home message for people with MS and their loved ones is that because the biochemical reactions occurring in MS are significantly different from those triggered in other autoimmune inflammatory diseases, treatment protocols may differ between diseases.

Speaking of triggers, let's take a closer look at some of the causes of neuroinflammation and the major mechanisms by which it occurs. We'll also examine some natural remedies and other pioneering approaches that hold promise as emerging therapies to address neuroinflammation and demyelination.

Neuroinflammation Triggers

Microglia are vulnerable to pro-inflammatory triggers such as stress, aging, diabetes, atherosclerosis, cardiovascular disease, obesity, and injury. As a result, those conditions are strongly associated with a higher risk of developing neurodegenerative diseases, the common thread for which is inflammation. For example, atherosclerosis—an arterial disease in which plaque builds up and causes a narrowing of the blood vessels—is a known source of vascular inflammation. Cardiovascular disease is strongly linked to inflammation as well. In fact, one of the key markers for identifying cardiovascular disease is elevated C-reactive protein (CRP), a marker for inflammation.

Having chronically high blood sugar levels, such as in type 2 diabetes, can trigger inflammation and is associated with significantly increased levels of beta-amyloid, the hallmark for Alzheimer's disease. Beta-amyloid is a sticky protein fragment that can accumulate and cause "plaques," or deposits of amyloid protein, in the brain. Amyloid plaques are thought to cause inflammation in the brain that blocks proper brain cell communication.

Obesity, which often accompanies cardiovascular disease and diabetes, is also known to be a chronically pro-inflammatory condition. All of these known inflammatory conditions are linked to increased risk not only of cognitive disorders and dementia, but also of other neurological conditions such as depression and anxiety.[15]

Nerve Growth Factor

Another interesting commonality among the inflammatory conditions previously mentioned is that they all are linked to having low levels of nerve growth factor (NGF): a neurotrophin, or growth factor protein, responsible for the development of neurons and the repair and regeneration of existing neurons. NGF controls the critical function of repairing the myelin sheath, the protective layer around axons that is damaged in MS. NGF has other seemingly unrelated actions, like protecting pancreatic cells and balancing immune and hormone activity. NGF may also help repair the heart after a heart attack and help rebuild damaged blood vessels.

Knowing how many systems are reliant on NGF, it must therefore be true that having high levels of NGF helps protect against neurodegenerative disease, right? Unfortunately, it's not that simple; in fact, it can actually be a case of too much of a good thing.

If that sounds contradictory, it's because NGF's story is a complicated one—and scientists acknowledge they still have so much to learn about it. For example, one of NGF's functions is to interact with the immune system via *mast cells*: white blood cells that release inflammatory compounds during allergic reactions, and which also appear in high numbers in some auto-immune conditions. Scientists have discovered that mast cells secrete NGF under certain conditions as part of their inflammatory response—but they don't fully understand why. Also, in certain autoimmune conditions such as rheumatoid arthritis, high levels of NGF are linked to a higher sensitivity to pain. Because of this correlation, pharmaceutical companies are developing and testing drugs that block or reduce NGF as a means of reducing pain.[16]

Since MS is also an autoimmune condition, perhaps it's not surprising that some patients also exhibit abnormally high NGF levels. Studies show that such levels can be found in the spinal cord fluid of MS patients who are experiencing high levels of pain and inflammation. High levels of inflammatory mast cells can be found in plaques residing in the brains of MS patients.[17] One small study demonstrated that MS patients with central neuropathic pain had much higher levels of NGF in their spinal fluid as compared with not only healthy people without MS, but also MS patients who were not experiencing pain.[18] Although not well understood, one interesting theory to explain the link between NGF and pain is that NGF is released in response to inflammation as a means of healing by regenerating damaged axons. But the consequence of healing the nerves is that pain perception becomes more acute.[19]

Despite the fact that high NGF levels are linked to inflammation and autoimmunity, it's still a beneficial compound for healing neurological damage related to MS. This is because it plays an important role in promoting remyelination. Research has shown that NGF can help delay the onset of MS, decrease neuroinflammation, repair myelin, and protect the brain. In our attempt to better understand the complexities of NGF, rather than labeling it as "good" or "bad," it may simply be a matter of balance. NGF is released by mast cells as an attempt for the body to heal, but that action can sometimes go too far. The excess NGF levels in MS may be a response to tissue damage, not the cause. Most likely, balanced levels of NGF are healthy and beneficial for the most part, but too low or too high is detrimental. Scientists may not have the exact answers yet, but it is clear that NGF has a positive impact on the nervous system under the right conditions and at the appropriate level, and in most cases it is beneficial to enhance NGF in a comprehensive MS treatment plan. See chapter 6 for more about NGF.

Stress

In a mouse study, stress induced by "repeated social defeat" triggered microglia to increase inflammatory signals in the brain.[20] In humans, chronic stress has been shown in many research studies to cause emotional disturbance, cognitive decline, and overall decline in mental health.[21] One such meta-analysis found "a consistent association between stressful life events and subsequent exacerbation in multiple sclerosis." However, it is important to realize that these data do not allow the linking of specific stressors to exacerbations, because most MS attacks are not related to stress. Nor should the study be used to infer that patients are responsible for their exacerbations. Investigation of the psychological, neuroendocrine, and immune mediators of stressful life events on exacerbation may lead to new behavioral and pharmacological strategies targeting potential links between stress and exacerbation.

Lack of Oxygen

A lack of adequate oxygen supply to the tissues of the body is called hypoxia. It is well known that hypoxia causes neuronal cell death, which is why a stroke can be so devastating. It also turns out that hypoxia can be a trigger for MS even in the absence of an autoimmune reaction: In other words, a deficit of oxygen can set up neuroinflammatory conditions that damage myelin even without involving the immune system. Studies show that prior to an MS attack that causes demyelination, there is a temporary reduction of oxygen in the CNS.[22] In one study using an animal model of MS to create neurological deficits, administering oxygen significantly restored function within an hour, and improvement persisted for at least seven days with continuous oxygen administration.[23]

Low oxygen levels also create a tremendously high burden of oxidation, a chemical process that itself causes neuronal cell death. On the other hand, if oxygen levels are high enough, animal studies have shown that demyelination can be prevented. This means that ensuring nerves have plenty of oxygen plays a crucial role in protecting neuronal health and preventing demyelination. (See also the "Oxidative Stress" section later in this chapter.)

Lack of Sleep

Sleep debt is a factor in weight gain, metabolic syndrome, and hormonal dysregulation, all factors that increase the risk of neurodegeneration.

Animal studies show that sleep deprivation causes activation of microglia and increased production of pro-inflammatory chemicals, which has a negative impact on memory and cognitive function. Poor sleep and irregular sleep patterns in humans increase microglial activity and promote the deposition of beta-amyloid protein plaques in the brain. Impaired sleep is associated with an increased risk of developing Alzheimer's disease.[24] Although impaired sleep is common among patients with MS, it hasn't so far been implicated as a cause of demyelination. I can attest that when I don't sleep enough, it affects my health in many ways. In chapters 8 and 9, I offer in-depth advice on how to achieve better sleep with supplements and lifestyle modifications.

Certain Infections

An abundance of published research shows that infection can trigger an immune response. This in turn can create neuroinflammation that can become neurodegenerative. Some viruses have been shown to directly damage neurons and cause neurodegeneration.[25] One study showed that chronic infection with cytomegalovirus (CMV) and certain herpes viruses (HSV), both of which take up latent but lifelong residency in the spinal cord, are linked with increased risk of neurodegeneration.[26] HSV has been shown in lab tests to increase production of amyloid proteins. Both viruses are associated with increased risk of cognitive decline. Bacterial infections, such as those caused by *H. pylori* and *Chlamydia*, are also implicated in an increased risk of Alzheimer's.[27]

In my experience, when I catch a common cold or flu, I'm much more likely to experience an MS relapse while I'm sick or shortly thereafter. Research studies confirm that my experience isn't unusual. One animal study showed that various influenza viruses had the ability to trigger neurological disease in autoimmune-prone mice.[28] Exposing these mice to various flu viruses caused clinical symptoms and pathological nerve damage. Other research shows that viral infections, such as in an upper respiratory infection, appear to activate the immune system, increase inflammation, and activate microglia to trigger neuroinflammation. Numerous human studies implicate viruses in triggering a relapse in MS and exacerbating inflammatory demyelination. MS patients who have a fever and flu-like symptoms not only are at risk for relapse, but also have much higher rates of hospitalization due to immune dysfunction.[29]

What about Vaccines?

You may be wondering, as I do: If infections as common as the flu can trigger a relapse in MS, then would it be beneficial to get a flu vaccination?

Many (but not all) studies support the value of vaccination for MS patients. One study reviewed a database of patients with primary progressive MS and evaluated the effects of vaccinations. Out of 180 patients experiencing MS relapse during the study, 33 percent had contracted the flu within the six weeks prior, whereas only 5 percent of patients who relapsed had received a vaccination.[30] From this study, it appeared that a relapse due to a vaccination reaction is much less probable than having a relapse due to contracting the flu.

Because infections can cause MS attacks and symptoms, it is important to avoid them or treat them as soon as possible. One of my tried-and-true methods for helping to ward off colds, flus, and other infections is fire cider, an old folk remedy and health tonic that is good for you and also happens to taste delicious.

Aging

Studies of older animals show that their microglia levels are higher, which means they have become both more sensitized to inflammatory conditions and more predisposed to experiencing inflammation. Similarly, in humans, the older adult brain contains more inflammatory microglia as well as more substances that provoke inflammation than are found in a younger brain.[31] Even an infection in another part of the body can trigger inflammation in the aging brain. And prolonged neuroinflammation has been shown to detrimentally affect memory and cognition.

Oxidative Stress

Oxidation is a chemical reaction related to the process of decomposition. Rust is an example of metal being oxidized, and when food is broken down

Fire Cider

This recipe, adapted from one by Mountain Rose Herbs, calls for infusing unfiltered, organic apple cider vinegar with a mixture of healthful ingredients, then straining the cider and adding honey to sweeten. I use it to both ward off and treat colds. You can experiment with other flavors to suit your liking.

½ cup freshly peeled and grated gingerroot

½ cup freshly grated horseradish root

1 medium onion, chopped

10 cloves garlic, crushed or chopped

2 organic jalapeño peppers, chopped

1 lemon, zest and juice

2 tablespoons dried rosemary leaves

1 tablespoon turmeric powder or 2 tablespoons freshly grated turmeric root

¼ teaspoon cayenne powder

Organic unfiltered apple cider vinegar

¼ cup raw honey, or to taste

1. Add the ginger, horseradish, onion, garlic, jalapeño peppers, lemon zest and juice, rosemary, turmeric, and cayenne powder into quart-sized glass jar.
2. Pour in apple cider vinegar until all the ingredients are fully covered and the vinegar reaches the top of the jar. You want to be sure all the ingredients are covered to prevent spoilage.
3. Use a piece of natural parchment paper under the lid to keep the vinegar from touching the metal, or use a plastic lid instead.
4. Shake the jar to combine all the ingredients and store in a dark, cool place for 4 to 6 weeks, remembering to shake the jar a few seconds every day.
5. After a month, use a mesh strainer or cheesecloth to strain out the solids, pouring the vinegar into a clean jar. Be sure to squeeze

out as much of the liquid as you can. This stuff is liquid gold! The solids can be used in a stir-fry, or you can compost/discard them.

6. Add honey to the liquid and stir until incorporated.
7. Taste your fire cider and add more honey if needed until you reach your desired sweetness.
8. Store in a sealed container in the refrigerator or in a cold, dark place.
9. Drink 1 to 2 tablespoons when needed.

into proteins, carbohydrates, and other basic units, it's due to oxidation. Cells rely on oxidative reactions to create energy. Normally this reaction is not detrimental, because it is balanced by antioxidant factors that counteract oxidative damage. But when oxidation becomes excessive, it creates high levels of reactive oxygen species (ROS)—reactive molecules that contain oxygen. High levels of ROS lead to oxidative stress. When ROS outweigh antioxidants, cells and tissues sustain damage. Oxidative stress has been shown to be a contributor to developing Parkinson's and Alzheimer's, and it's also known to be a major contributor to multiple sclerosis progression by inducing demyelination and axonal damage.

Oxidation is closely linked with inflammation.[32] The inflammatory process generates high levels of oxidizing radicals, causing further damage. Oxidation impacts the immune system and accelerates the progression of autoimmune disorders including MS. Inflammation activates the recruitment of immune cells such as T cells, microglia, and macrophages to the lesion sites, causing further demyelination of the nerves.

Oxidative factors also contribute to lesions in the brains of MS patients, as the DNA in neuronal cells become oxidized and damaged. Oxidation contributes to telomere shortening, which accelerates aging and disease progression. Telomeres are the protective caps at the end of DNA strands, somewhat like the protective seal on the tip of a shoelace that prevents it from unraveling. Long telomeres are protective to cells, and short telomeres signify that the cell is not protected and is near the end of its life span. Short telomeres are associated with aging, increased risk of cancer, and even death. Some research suggests that oxidative stress leads to increased inflammation, which ultimately damages telomeres and causes them to shorten. Studies have compared telomere length in MS patients with that in healthy controls, and found that telomere length was significantly shorter in patients with PPMS (primary progressive MS) than in people who are healthy or have less severe MS.

Measuring oxidative status may be a way to quantify the degree to which neuroinflammation and neurodegenerative disease have progressed. SOD, superoxide dismutase, is an important defensive antioxidative enzyme produced in the body that can be measured. SOD activity has been shown to be lower in MS patients who have more severe disability, as determined by more radiological lesions and longer disease duration. Studies also show higher levels of oxidative compounds in cases of more severe disability.

To reinforce the importance of counteracting oxidative stress, one study demonstrated that patients with MS who have a less severe disease course had much higher levels of antioxidant factors such as coenzyme Q10 (CoQ10) compared with patients who had more progressed MS. Studies also suggest that many women with MS do not consume enough antioxidant and anti-inflammatory nutrients like quercetin and magnesium. Eating a diet with an abundance of vegetables and fruits helps ensure high levels of antioxidants, which potentially slow or halt MS progression.[33]

Particulate matter in the air (air pollution) is another potential, though as yet unproven, immune trigger for MS relapse. There has been very little research, but one specific study conducted in Europe found that seasonally elevated levels of particulate matter caused an increased risk of relapse for MS patients. Researchers think this may be due to increased oxidative stress.[34]

An Altered Microbiome

And here we've come full circle.

As I mentioned earlier in this chapter, the gut-brain axis comprises a highly complex, bidirectional communication system that regulates multiple neurochemical and neurometabolic pathways that connect the GI tract, skin, liver, and other organs with both the enteric and central nervous systems, including the brain—and influences endocrine, immune, nervous, and other physiological systems operations.

Although the GBA's exact mechanisms remain under investigation, studies have shown that—just as neurological stress can affect the microbiome—an altered microbiome can cause pathologies within the brain.

Let's dig in a little here. Much like the intestinal barrier, the blood-brain barrier (BBB) is a highly selective, semipermeable membrane within the capillaries of the brain—where endothelial tight junctions (very close spaces between the cells lining the capillaries) serve as gatekeepers, allowing only particular substances such as fat-soluble molecules and certain gases *in*, while keeping pathogens and toxins *out*. However, in studies of laboratory mice, researchers discovered that, by releasing specific materials into the bloodstream, a leaky gut can lead to increased permeability within the blood-brain barrier.[35]

A 2014 study demonstrates the overall ramifications of this. In investigating the possible links between dysbiosis and Parkinson's disease (an inflammatory neurological disease), researchers determined that the hallmarks of Parkinson's—known as Lewy bodies and Lewy neurons—are actually "primed" in the gut.[36] According to this model, the process involves normal proteins called alpha-synucleins (α-synucleins), which are abundant in the brain and present in smaller numbers elsewhere in the body. While the function of α-synucleins isn't well understood, scientists believe they're implicated in transmitting messages across nerve synapses.

During their research, investigators discovered that α-synucleins become damaged—or misfolded—in the intestinal tract due to toxins or other microbiome imbalances. They then travel to the brain via the vagus nerve, where they begin to inflict harm upon healthy neurons. In other words, a damaged blood-brain barrier, triggered by dysbiosis, is complicit in the development of Parkinson's disease. Researchers have also discovered that specific imbalances in the gut—namely, a proliferation of harmful pathogens in the Enterobacteriaceae family (gram-negative bacteria including *Salmonella*, *E. coli*, and *Shigella*, among others), and/or a deficiency of helpful microbes in the Prevotellaceae family (also gram-negative bacteria, often found in the digestive tracts of those whose diets are low in animal fats)—are correlated with a higher risk for, and severity of, Parkinson's.[37]

As it turns out, the same may be true for Alzheimer's disease. Studies have shown that as individuals age, both the gut's epithelial barrier and the blood-brain barrier become increasingly more permeable—likely due to cumulative environmental and other external influences, including chronic infections and low-fiber, high-sugar diets. In turn, this exposes the CNS to neurotoxins that take up residence in the brain and begin damaging neurons and cells in ways that are associated with the disease. For example, certain opportunistic fungal and yeast infections of the CNS—enabled via a compromised microbiome-gut-brain-axis—are correlated with increased risk for Alzheimer's. (Research has shown that the surface structures of these invaders promote the development of amyloid protein, a hallmark of the disease, in the brain.[38])

Similarly, when herpes simplex virus (HSV-1—which often establishes lifelong latency in the CNS of infected individuals) infects human brain cells, molecules called inflammatory cytokines concentrate in areas of the brain where amyloid plaques have developed. This suggests, at the very least, a correlation between the virus entering the brain via a compromised barrier, resulting neuroinflammation, and the development of Alzheimer's.[39]

In addition, there's a study linking specific prions (normal proteins that, for a variety of reasons, mutate and self-replicate) with the development of several neurodegenerative diseases, including Alzheimer's, Parkinson's, and amyotrophic lateral sclerosis (ALS, or Lou Gehrig's disease). According to researchers, who note that the risk for many neurodegenerative diseases increases with age (there's that leaky gut and damaged blood-brain barrier again!), these prions aggregate into tangles in the brain that lead to pathology. In the case of Alzheimer's, researchers postulate that such prions serve as receptors for the amyloid-beta (Aβ) peptides that ultimately make up the disease's characteristic amyloid fibrils.

But how do those prions reach the brain? This is where it gets interesting. In a separate study in laboratory mice, scientists demonstrated that injected prions arrive there from elsewhere in the body, presumably through the blood-brain barrier, where they cause neuroinflammation, synaptic degeneration, and amyloidogenesis. While more research is necessary, it remains well within the realm of possibility that dysbiosis is among the likely culprits for these prions' ability to enter the brain.

Stress hormones also seem to play a role in cognitive impairment. Researchers have discovered that "germ-free" mice—those that effectively lack a microbiome—experience higher-than-normal activity in the hypothalamic-pituitary-adrenal (HPA) axis, a major neuroendocrine system that controls not only the body's reaction to stress but also several other biological processes including mood and emotion.[40] When activity in the HPA axis is elevated, corticosterone—a stress hormone manufactured in the adrenal glands—similarly rises. And, according to a study published in the journal *Neuroscience*, "chronic exposure to . . . corticosterone is known to alter plasticity within hippocampal and amygdalar circuits that mediate fear learning and memory."[41] In other words, an imbalanced microbiome leads to a hyperactive HPA axis, causing symptoms of increased anxiety, difficulties with spatial learning, and memory impairment.

Additionally, increased levels of corticotropin-releasing hormone (CRH)—the main engine behind HPA axis functioning—have been shown to trigger anxiety and clinical depression. As scientists understand it, high levels of CRH first disrupt the microbiome and cause leaky gut. Endotoxins are released into the bloodstream, stimulating the body's immune response, which inhibits secretion of neurotransmitters such as serotonin and the catecholamines (dopamine, epinephrine, and norepinephrine, among others). Decreased levels of these neurotransmitters are associated with memory impairments and autism spectrum disorders (ASDs).

And there's more. We also know that endotoxins, such as lipopolysaccharides (LPSs) from bacteria, or polysaccharides from *Candida*, can easily escape a leaky gut and release a variety of cytokines (chemical messengers) into the bloodstream—a process that drives a sudden, acute inflammatory reaction: one that's been implicated in blood-brain barrier disruption. Comprising fats (lipids) and sugar, LPSs are both structural to, and protective of, normally benign bacteria. When those bacteria die, the LPSs are released into the surrounding environment with little effect or fanfare. In the presence of a leaky gut, however, the story is different.

According to research, investigators have stimulated neuroinflammation in mice by injecting LPSs directly into the animals' abdomens.[42] In turn, this resulted in memory loss and increased brain levels of beta-amyloid—a factor implicated in Alzheimer's disease. LPSs can also play a role in the course and severity of demyelinating diseases such as autoimmune encephalomyelitis (EAE). In fact, researchers studying MS mimic this in animals by using LPSs to induce EAE.

But how, exactly, does leaky gut occur? We touched on it a little earlier; more specifically, it starts with the intestinal lining itself—and a molecule called zonulin.

Zonulin is responsible for regulating the tight junctions of the intestinal barrier. Serving as a physiological gatekeeper, it allows the passage of good molecules, such as nutrients, from the gut into the bloodstream, where they can be absorbed. However, when damaging factors deregulate this so-called zonulin pathway, normally unacceptable molecules can slip through—where they can potentially cause an unwelcome immune response in genetically susceptible individuals.[43] Interestingly, MS patients are known to have higher serum levels of zonulin, which places them at higher risk for leaky gut and immune reactions.

Considered together with additional evidence linking imbalances in the gut to memory and cognitive impairments, this research holds fascinating promise for better understanding and treating many neurological diseases— including multiple sclerosis.

If you've been following along, you won't be surprised that dysbiosis and its effects—like neuroinflammation, above, and immune system dysfunction, below—play a prominent role in the disease. Numerous studies back this up. Thanks to the power of DNA analysis, for example, we know that certain single-celled organisms, such as *Methanobrevibacter* and *Akkermansia*, proliferate in our guts, while bacteria like *Lactobacillus*, *Coprobacillus*, and *Haemophilus* appear in much smaller numbers than in the general population.

It's pretty clear, then, that dysbiosis and leaky gut can be bad news for the brain—especially if these conditions remain uncorrected. The *good* news, however, is that many of these neurological impairments appear to be *reversible*. And they begin with your lifestyle. (I'll discuss this in greater detail in chapter 5.)

Dysbiosis and Mitochondrial Dysfunction

One of the effects of dysbiosis is damage to mitochondria. I hesitate to highlight mitochondrial dysfunction as a discrete topic. On the one hand, it is closely linked to neuroinflammation. But on the other, researchers have yet to determine whether there's a cause-and-effect relationship between the two. Still, I believe its role in MS is important enough to call out, even if we don't fully understand it yet.

Mitochondria are responsible for a variety of biochemical reactions in the body, but they're best known as the powerhouses of cells because of their role in producing adenosine triphosphate (ATP), which the body uses for energy. A necessary part of producing energy involves creating substances known as free radicals. You've probably heard of free radicals as causes of oxidative stress. Under normal circumstances, the body can protect the mitochondria and other cells from damage caused by oxidative stress by activating its own antioxidant systems. This process, which allows mitochondria to function optimally, is a beautiful example of how our bodies are designed to work within a dynamic balance. When this balance is impaired for some reason, mitochondria may become damaged and produce even more free-radical substances, thereby creating a vicious cycle of increasing cellular damage from excess oxidation.[44]

The central nervous system has a high demand for energy, which makes it especially vulnerable to the effects of mitochondrial dysfunction. Damaged mitochondria have been detected in axons and neurons in the white matter of the brain in both people with MS and animal models of MS.

Dysfunctional mitochondria appear to be a major contributor to the progression of MS. This may help explain why pharmaceutical treatments aimed at reducing neuroinflammation haven't been effective at halting disease progression—because they don't address the underlying mitochondrial dysfunction. Mitochondrial dysfunction is also present in other neurodegenerative diseases, such as Alzheimer's, Parkinson's, and Huntington's. There is still much to learn about the role of mitochondrial damage in neurodegeneration, but it is clearly an important aspect of MS progression that needs to be targeted in future research.

————

You might be wondering, "All this knowledge is fascinating, but what does it mean to *me*?" The answer is: Quite a bit, because the more we understand how the microbiome contributes to the immune system, and how an unhealthy microbiome can contribute to neurological damage, the better we can counteract that damage using some simple strategies. In fact, it's around such knowledge that I've designed, personally tested, and refined my own comprehensive treatment plan. The good news is that it is possible to prevent dysbiosis with commonsense, easy-to-follow strategies. In doing so, you can ameliorate the symptoms of MS, as I will illustrate through my own personal experience.

Your ultimate goal is to create, support, and sustain a healthy microbiome, because if you can remove the conditions that lead to leaky gut, neuroinflammation, immune dysfunction, and a compromised gut-brain axis, you can not only protect against demyelination but even encourage remyelination.

CHAPTER 4

Returning to the Jungle

I traveled to Ecuador five times, and participated in over 60 ceremonies with Juan Uyunkar and his family. Partly because I was a student of the plants and ceremonies, and partly because of wellness, I appreciated that Juan was willing to share his culture with me. At the time of my visits, I had been experiencing disease symptoms that included frequent urination, occasional muscle spasms, sleep apnea, and subtle breathing irregularities. I had no idea that these symptoms might be serious—or that they were symptoms of MS.

Juan lived near Quito, Ecuador's capital, with his many children and his wife, Rosa, a jeweler. Juan was a traditional medicine man, but he also lived a modern life: used a cell phone, drove a car, and loved pop movies. Once, Juan and I were in the jungle far away from any people, gathering plants that he used to make poison for applying to arrows during hunting. His cell phone rang! It was his family, asking him how his summer was going.

He spoke in combinations of Spanish and Shuar, and performed ceremonies using what's known as natem, the traditional herbal preparation that the Shuar use to heal. All his family partook, even his reluctant kids. The children fasted, took herbs, then vomited and had visions after praying. (The visions were not hallucinations caused by the herbs, but arose from a series of ceremonial processes.)

Taking Out the Trash

After listening to my story and sitting with me in ceremonies, Juan told me my problem was that I was full of garbage. (Later, I realized this was what he told almost everyone.) His standard treatment for disease was to *vacía la basura*, or empty the garbage, from the gut. To do this, I would use natem, too.

Juan made clear that he would not want to share natem with "hippies who like drugs," because this is not the purpose of taking these sacred plants. In addition, he pointed out that the Shuar natem should not be confused with *ayahuasca* from Peru, an herbal blend that includes leaves of a psychoactive herb called chacruna (*Psychotria viridis*). In fact, Juan considers the other psychoactive blends of what Westerners think of as ayahuasca as neurotoxins that he would never consider using or offering.

The natem ceremony usually involves consuming a tea brewed from a combination of the vine *Banisteriopsis caapi* and two other leaves that contain potent alkaloids. Over three days practitioners mix a large batch of these herbs with water and boil it until the liquid condenses into a small bottle of thick, molasses-like syrup.

Juan explained that the preparation was designed to have little to no hallucinogenic effect, but that its purgative element would be strong: I would experience severe vomiting and diarrhea throughout the process as the "garbage" was expelled from my system. As I drank the thick syrup, my whole body shuddered. And its effect on my digestive system was exactly as Juan said it would be: excessive purgation, over a period of three days.

While the natem treatments provided some level of resolution for my symptoms and increased my vitality, the symptoms did not completely disappear, and my condition remained undiagnosed. But after being diagnosed with multiple sclerosis, I would return to the idea of cleansing the gut as a treatment, because it had made me feel lighter and more energetic.

Many practitioners recommend treating the gut ecosystem with oral probiotics—supplements that add beneficial bacteria to the microbiome. Unfortunately, changing the microbiome is not that simple. There isn't much evidence that oral probiotics can successfully inoculate the gut with a new microbiome to the extent that is required. Diets that induce a healthy microbiome, such as avoiding all sugars and eating a variety of fiber-rich, whole, and fermented foods, are a more viable path to changing the composition of the microbiome, but this method can take many years to accomplish the goal.

Although the human microbiome first developed 50,000 years ago, our understanding of it remains quite primitive. Plus, given all the dietary and environmental factors involved, it would be nearly impossible for humans to re-create the optimal microbiome with a pill or potion. If you're interested in altering your own microbiome as part of your MS treatment plan, as I have, the best option available today is to undergo a fecal microbial transplant from a healthy donor.

My Experience with Fecal Microbial Transplant

Fecal microbial transplant (FMT) is a procedure in which feces from a healthy donor is processed and tested and then inserted via catheter into another person's colon. The transplanted material normally contains 50 trillion colony-forming units (CFUs) per dose with over 1,000 different species per *healthy* donor. By contrast, a commercially available oral probiotic pill usually contains only millions or billions of CFUs, representing only a dozen or so different species.

Fecal transplant treatments are administered after a GI lavage such as a colonic or a purging enema to release as many bacteria from the colon as possible. It can be administered once daily for a sequence of days. The more doses administered, the better chance of recolonizing a new microbiome. Some clinics recommend 1 day of treatment; others recommend 10 days. Because it's a new type of treatment, the recommended numbers of treatments have not yet been standardized.

Fecal transplant works well to treat *Clostridium difficile* (*C. diff*), a bacterium that can gain a foothold in the gut after damage to the microbiota caused by antibiotics. *C. diff* infection produces symptoms including chronic diarrhea and severe inflammation of the colon. Endotoxins produced by *Clostridium* disrupt the blood-brain barrier, making it permeable to cytokines and causing neuroinflammation. At almost 90 percent, fecal transplants have an astounding cure rate for *C. diff* infections.

Treatment with fecal transplant has also been shown to have an effect on multiple sclerosis. In a study published in the *American Journal of Gastroenterology* in 2011, Australian gastroenterologist Dr. Thomas Borody and his associates reported that, as a possible treatment for constipation, they had performed FMT therapy on three wheelchair-bound MS patients.

Unsurprisingly to the researchers, the patients' bowel symptoms resolved following FMT; what *did* surprise them were the unexpected side benefits of FMT. Two of the patients, both of whom had previously required indwelling urinary catheters, experienced restoration of their urinary function. Remarkably, all three patients regained their ability to walk unassisted. In one patient of the three, a follow-up MRI taken 15 years after FMT showed a halting of disease progression and "no evidence of active disease."[1]

After I read this report, I decided to explore a fecal microbial transplant for myself. At that time, the only clinic that offered FMT to patients not suffering from *C. diff* was located in the Bahamas. My doctor, Bill Cody, MD, who also has primary progressive MS, recommended the Taymount Clinic.

Dr. Cody had undergone a variety of treatments, including FMT, and had successfully progressed from using a wheelchair to walking independently. I had also watched a YouTube video of an MS patient similar to myself in age and symptomology. He had responded well to FMT therapy for his constipation, and his ability to walk also improved. I read about another MS patient, too, whose constipation had resolved after just two FMT therapies.

Based on these inspirational stories, I decided to go to the Taymount, where I became part of a clinical trial that assessed patient outcomes of FMT therapy for a variety of chronic diseases, including MS. The protocol of the study was quite simple: Go to the sunny Bahamas, receive a series of FMT therapies, follow up with 10 more at-home treatments over the next six months, and track my symptoms throughout.

I hoped that, at a minimum, my participation might help with at least one of my chronic symptoms: the severe constipation that had developed four years prior during an MS attack. In conventional medicine's view, the bowel problems that MS patients experience are simply due to demyelination—it doesn't acknowledge that the microbiome's balance, or lack thereof, might be a contributing factor.

During the first week of treatment, I was disappointed that my constipation didn't improve. The doctors told me to be patient. "It takes at least three months to restore the gut flora," they said, suggesting that my symptoms might change within that time frame.

As they predicted, changing my microbiome did significantly impact my gastrointestinal health in terms of digestion over time. My constipation decreased about 30 percent. Six months after going to the Bahamas, other symptoms improved even more significantly: paresthesia, Lhermitte's syndrome (the feeling of electric shock experienced when bending the neck), fatigue, sleepiness, and cognitive impairment all changed for the better. Overall, the total of my symptoms decreased by 50 percent, and when my neurologist tested my neurocognitive index, my results indicated dramatic improvements in attention, memory, problem solving, and my ability to identify and recognize almost every human emotion—except bad ones!

Repairing the Microbiome

If the microbiome plays a critical role in the development and progression of MS, then repairing that microbiome is critical to slowing or halting the disease in its tracks. It may even prevent the disease in the first place.

Every day, we learn more about how critical the microbiome is to human health. As we've seen, it plays a special role in MS and other autoimmune diseases, and is likely implicated in many other conditions as well. Although fecal microbial transplant is a fast and dramatic way to alter the microbiome's bacterial makeup, the time and cost involved means it isn't the most ideal—or practical—solution for many MS patients.

Fortunately, as I have learned during my time as a naturopathic physician, and throughout my own multiple sclerosis journey, there are many ways in which diet and dietary supplements can support a healthy microbiome. Two simple, easy-to-follow strategies you can follow to get yours into optimal shape are to increase the diversity of your diet and to be sure your diet includes plenty of certain types of carbohydrate called *prebiotics*.

Widen Your Dietary (and Microbial) Diversity

In chapter 2 I quoted the adage, "the only people who get sick are the ones who leave the jungle." The reasons why people who leave traditional natural indigenous lifestyles for the modern industrialized world begin suffering from chronic degenerative diseases include chemical exposure, environmental toxins, processed food, and stress. But a primary reason may relate to changes in the microbiome when people engage with modern industrialized culture.

Indigenous people living a traditional natural lifestyle mostly avoid diseases such as irritable bowel syndrome, heart disease, diabetes, and even MS. Why? Because, they host a much greater diversity of microbial species in their guts. One reason for this is their dietary diversity.

Some gut bacteria have very specific nutritional needs that—if unmet—will result in those bacteria dying off. In Western culture the contemporary diet often focuses on a small number of staple goods that, thanks to refrigeration, transportation infrastructure, and commercial grocery chains, are available year-round. Therefore, because Westerners' diets are much less diverse than those of traditional indigenous peoples, so, too, are their microbiomes.

Despite what the Paleo diet's name implies, it's not possible for urban and suburban dwellers to simply copy the diet of aboriginal peoples. (For more on this diet and its many benefits, see the "Paleo Diet" section in chapter 5.) But it *is* possible to diversify the gut's bacteria and nourish the microbiome with foods that keep helpful bacteria healthy.

While I was undergoing my fecal microbial transplant, the Taymount Clinic's staff provided a simple tracking sheet to help me increase my dietary variety. I've found it to be an invaluable long-term tool—and it's one that anyone can easily adopt. Organized weekly, the sheet included 50 blank spaces in which I could record the foods I ate. My goal was to hit all 50, without repeating any foods, by the end of the week. Meats, grains, vegetables—even oils, herbs, and spices—counted. Bread would be counted once, no matter its form. I didn't always meet my 50-item goal, but the chart helped me achieve the diversity I needed to keep my microbiome healthy.

Concentrate on Prebiotics

Prebiotics comprise specific fibers and complex carbohydrates that human digestive enzymes can't break down—but that microorganisms in the gut can. When microbes break down insoluble fibers from plant matter and carbs via fermentation, they convert those fibers to acetate, propionate, and butyrate. These compounds are called short-chain fatty acids (SCFAs)—the main source of energy for cells that line the colon.[2] Researchers believe that SCFAs play a role in preventing certain cancers, inflammatory diseases, metabolic syndrome, and bowel disorders. SCFAs also influence energy regulation in the body.[3]

Including prebiotics in your diet can help your microbiome thrive—but only if your gut is already populated with good flora. (Adding prebiotics to the diet is not advisable for those whose gut flora is in poor condition; it may worsen problems with gas and indigestion.) In general, concentrate on consuming the following types of prebiotics, which are available in whole foods as well as commercial supplements. There are many options; there's no need to be overly concerned about which ones to choose. To start off, try cooking with lots of garlic and onions and leeks. If you try a new prebiotic and it doesn't agree with you, then stop using it. For example, I tried Jerusalem artichokes and found that I can't digest them, so I don't eat them anymore.

Fructo-Oligosaccharides (FOSs)

Foods high in FOSs include onions, spring onions, garlic, leeks, chickpeas, watermelon, tomatoes, asparagus, Jerusalem artichoke, globe artichoke, wheat, barley, honey, banana, dandelion leaves, dandelion root, and burdock root.

Inulin

Similar to FOS, inulin is highly concentrated in dandelion root, chicory root, and Jerusalem artichokes. It's also found in globe artichokes, asparagus, leeks, onions, bananas, wheat, maize, rice, and garlic.

Arabinogalactan

You can find this complex fiber in carrots, radishes, pears, corn, wheat, sorghum, black gram beans, fresh turmeric root, tomatoes, coconut meat, coconut flour, and even red wine. One of its primary sources, however, is the larch tree—so this is a prebiotic most often taken in supplemental form.

Beta-Glucans

These polysaccharides are present in grains such as oats and barley, and in mushrooms, seaweeds, and *Saccharomyces cerevisiae* (brewers' yeast). Beta glucans are often taken in supplemental form and are also known to support the health of the immune system.

Polyphenols

Polyphenols are naturally occurring compounds found in a variety of plant foods including fruits, vegetables, tea, coffee, chocolate, and wine. Because they act like prebiotics in the gut, polyphenols are another good food source for the microbiome. Like prebiotic fibers, gut bacteria will ferment polyphenols and produce SCFAs. Rich sources of polyphenols include: spices and herbs, berries, tea, cocoa, dark chocolate, ground flaxseeds, chestnuts, pecans, almonds (skin on), and many other plant foods.

CHAPTER 5

Putting Out the Fire of Neuroinflammation

Inflammation is the body's normal, healthy response to injury and invasion, and is critical to the process of healing. But when it becomes chronic, it can also wreak all sorts of havoc throughout the body, from the joints (arthritis) to the arteries (heart disease) and everything in between. And as I've explained in previous chapters, inflammation in its most insidious forms can also lead to neurodegenerative diseases like MS.

The good news is, many forms of chronic inflammation are related to our modern lifestyle and are therefore well within our ability to control. While those of us with MS can't turn back the clock and prevent ourselves from getting the disease, we *can* significantly reduce its daily impacts by addressing the root causes of neuroinflammation. Which brings me back to my favorite mantra: Your lifestyle is your best medicine.

In this chapter I'll discuss how changing—or improving upon—specific lifestyle factors, including diet, exercise, and nutritional supplementation, can successfully ease inflammation throughout the body.

Exercise

Exercise may not be the first thing you think of for supporting the brain, but in reviewing the research, it becomes clear that exercise is an essential component of a treatment protocol to prevent or slow the progression of neurodegenerative disorders.[1]

The benefits of exercise to the central nervous system (CNS) are outstanding, especially in relationship to neuroinflammation. It's well known that physical activity improves cardiovascular endurance, enhances muscle tone and strength, and improves metabolism to help moderate weight. It also has psychological benefits, and is recommended as part of a treatment protocol for depression and schizophrenia because of its mood-enhancing effects. But exercise also helps prevent neurodegeneration because it modulates the immune system and reduces inflammation.[2] Clinical studies demonstrate that physical activity reduces the risk of developing neurodegenerative disease, and slows the progression of cognitive decline turning into Alzheimer's disease (AD). Studies show that regular exercise can reduce the risk of developing AD by almost threefold![3]

More Ways Exercise Is Good for the Brain

Exercise is also one of several factors that can improve neuroplasticity to help overcome neurodegeneration in the aging brain. Neuroplasticity is the ability of the brain to learn new behaviors and rewire itself by making new neural connections. Caloric restriction, transcranial magnetic stimulation, deep brain stimulation, and even some medications can improve neuroplasticity.[4]

Animal studies show that exercise enhances neuroplasticity through enhanced dopamine production, increased blood flow to the brain, and neurotransmitter balance. Not all forms of exercise are equal; skill-based exercise affects different parts of the brain than does simple aerobic exercise through repetitive movement (say, an exercise bike). Aerobic exercise includes any activity that enhances oxygen use and circulation, whereas skilled exercise such as playing soccer uses spatial skills and has goal-oriented movement. Both types have unique positive effects on the brain and neuroplasticity. Exercises that involve both skill and aerobics, such as swimming or running, may have a synergistic effect, offering the maximum benefits for enhancing neuroplasticity.[5]

A review of research studying the impact of exercise on cognitively impaired patients discovered that the risk of developing dementia is as much as 35 percent lower in adults who are physically active as compared with those who are sedentary.[6] Aerobics and strength training, combined, were shown to have the most beneficial effects on cognitive function, particularly working memory and attention.

A review of the extensive amount of research on exercise shows that it impacts the immune system via several pathways. Multiple studies show that it can reduce a variety of pro-inflammatory cytokines that induce inflammation throughout the body. (For more specifics on how pro-inflammatory cytokines exert their influence, please refer to the "Dysbiosis and Neuroinflammation" section of chapter 3.)

When it comes to exercise, it's important to remember that moderation, rather than overexertion, is the goal—especially for MS patients. The Multiple Sclerosis Society of Canada offers guidelines for exercise, recommending 30 minutes of moderate aerobic activity, twice per week, plus strength-training exercises for major muscle groups twice per week.[7] These moderate exercise recommendations are intended for MS patients with relapsing-remitting or progressive forms, with minimal to moderate disability. The National Multiple Sclerosis Society offers a brochure titled "Exercise as Part of Everyday Life," which offers instructive exercises that focus on moderation.[8] Moderation is especially important for MS patients; besides the negative consequences to the immune system, there is the risk of overheating, and MS patients are particularly vulnerable to overheating, which can lead to worsened nerve conduction, increased fatigue, blurred vision, or impaired balance. Aqua exercise is an ideal choice for avoiding overheating, and it makes movement much easier. Strength training can be done with weight machines or resistance exercises. Recommendations advise starting with low weights and building up slowly, taking at least one day of recovery in between sessions. Yoga is an excellent choice for exercise; it can help stretch and strengthen muscles and enhances respiratory function. Exercise regimes that incorporate balance are especially helpful to counteract the neurological damage caused by MS pathology, and consistent practice can help train the brain and muscles to compensate for any weak areas. Aerobic exercise should be incorporated, and can be done in as little as five-minute increments, increased gradually to build up endurance. Essentially any type of movement is beneficial, and focusing on enjoyment will make you more likely to exercise regularly.

Diet

One of the most impactful triggers of inflammation in the body is the food we put in our mouths. But the range of diet recommendations for limiting inflammation can be difficult to figure out.

Choosing foods carefully is so important, because so many foods can potentially contribute to neuroinflammation.

Sugar is right at the top of this list. Processed sugar and refined carbohydrates trigger the release of pro-inflammatory cytokines. On average, Americans consume almost 66 pounds of added sugar per year, or about 82 grams per day.[9] The World Health Organization recommends only 25 grams per day, but that's less than the amount in a serving of the leading brand of yogurt—so much for considering yogurt to be a healthy snack! Sugar is hidden in salad dressings, white bread, packaged cereals, condiments, beverages, and much more. Be sure to check the labels of all packaged and processed foods before you eat them. As research has widely shown, and as the general public is becoming more and more aware, high-fructose corn syrup (which is metabolized differently from sucrose and is linked to obesity and inflammation) is one of the worst forms of sugar and should be avoided entirely.

Consuming excess added sugar also has a multiplying effect: The more we eat, the more our body craves it. In fact, studies show that sugar consumption triggers changes in the brain that resemble alcohol or drug addiction.[10]

Many types of anti-inflammatory diets exist, and they all have certain principles in common. They each recommend:

- Including oils and fats that are high in polyunsaturated fatty acids (PUFAs) like fish, flaxseed, and sunflower oil.
- Eating more nuts and seeds.
- Avoiding refined carbohydrates such as sugar (of all kinds) and honey.

- Avoiding trans fats, which are found in fried foods, pastries, margarine, and other processed food products. (Trans fats may appear on product labels as partially hydrogenated oils.)

Polyunsaturated fatty acids (PUFAs) can be tricky: They include omega-3 and -6 oils, which are also called omega-3 or omega-6 fatty acids or fats. Because omega-6 fats have the potential to be inflammatory when they are not in balance with omega-3 fats, they should be consumed with this in mind. Oils high in omega-6 include corn oil, safflower, sunflower, peanut, and vegetable oils. (Americans generally consume too much omega-6 oil, which is why I personally advise trying to scale it back in your diet and focus more on consuming more omega-3s.) Gluten, which is present in wheat, barley, and rye grains, and casein, a specific protein found in most dairy products, are both common allergens. (Gluten can also trigger celiac disease, a relatively rare autoimmune condition, in those who carry the gene for it.) Not everyone experiences issues with gluten and casein, of course, but because they can escalate inflammation in those who are sensitive, some anti-inflammatory diets exclude them.

Research on Dietary Intervention

Patients with multiple sclerosis are highly likely to turn to dietary modifications as a means of helping control their disease and feeling more empowered. Yet a 2012 Cochrane review of dietary interventions for MS research concluded that diet did not have a significant effect on MS disease progression or risk of clinical relapse.[11] (Cochrane is a nonprofit, independent organization that promotes evidence-based health care decision making.) That may cause patients to feel less hopeful about trying diet therapy. Please don't be discouraged by this, because diet has been shown to increase quality of life and symptoms of fatigue in MS, and an ongoing study of the impact of the Wahls diet on MS looks promising. It's important to keep in mind that there were significant limitations to the Cochrane review. The most important was their inclusion criteria, which were fairly limited: Out of 923 published studies related to diet and supplementation for treating MS, only 6 randomized studies qualified for their review. All six of those studies were focused on PUFAs, specifically omega-3 and -6 supplementation. The remaining 917 studies, which focused on diverse diet topics such as hypoallergenic diets and nutrient supplementation, were excluded because they did not meet their design criteria. The reasons for exclusion varied, such as because a study wasn't randomized (meaning that the treatment group was not compared with a control group within the study) or because the study endpoints did not match those as defined by the Cochrane inclusion criteria. The Cochrane study conclusion was therefore limited to just a review of the role of dietary fats in treating MS. Despite this fact, the study's overall determination was that dietary interventions are not clinically therapeutic for treating MS, and that MS patients should simply follow general healthy diet guidelines.

This determination ignores the reality of dietary intervention: Unlike pharmaceutical research on a single chemical compound, research on the effects of ingesting a single food or a single nutrient rarely shows significant results. This is because an effective nutritional protocol needs to be broad and comprehensive, including a synergy of foods, nutrients, and lifestyle adjustments. In this Cochrane review, the inclusion criteria were too limited for dietary intervention research. It included less than 1 percent of existing studies on dietary interventions, and thus a plethora of useful information was overlooked.

Polyunsaturated Fatty Acids

Historically, dietary fats have gotten a bad rap in the media, but current research indicates that certain categories of fats are not only healthy but also essential for critical functions, including brain and nerve cell membrane growth and development; hormone synthesis; neurotransmitter synthesis; cell membrane formation; and much more.[12]

Topping the list of healthy fats are omega-3s, which can only be acquired through diet and supplementation. Omega-3 fats include the subgroups docosahexaenoic acid (DHA) and eicosapentaenoic acid (EPA). Although the Cochrane review did not support the use of omega-3 fats for treating MS, many other studies indicate that these healthy fats can provide benefits, including reducing inflammatory markers and the rates of disease relapse. They may even reduce the effects of fatigue and depression, which improves patients' overall quality of life.[13]

Remember also that when you consume omega-3 fats through the food you eat, you're ingesting a much more complex array (and sometimes a larger quantity) of beneficial nutrients than a simple supplement can provide. I think this is a major reason why research on PUFAs, which generally is limited to testing single supplements that contain single ingredients, has not shown positive results. It is much more difficult to conduct a research study on real food, because any single whole food contains so many constituents. There are too many factors that cannot be controlled for, which is something that researchers hate!

DHA and EPA are present in higher levels in the brain than in other parts of the body and are both critical for fetus and infant brain development. Research has shown that EPA deficiency in early development can cause poor myelination in the brain and lower cognitive function.[14] High-dose omega-3 intake is shown to be beneficial in neurodegenerative and neurological diseases and to balance mood disorders. DHA is a nutritional cofactor in nerve membrane development, specifically in the sphingomyelin—a phosphate-containing fatty acid found in the myelin sheath. Low DHA alters spatial memory and neurotransmission.

Omega-3 fatty acids (both EPA and DHA) play a significant role in decreasing neuroinflammation by inhibiting pro-inflammatory cytokine production and altering specific biochemical pathways in an anti-inflammatory direction.[15] Research shows that people who have higher serum levels of EPA (compared with a control group) have a lower risk of developing pathologies of the brain (including gray matter atrophy, a common sign in MS related to cognitive impairment) and a lower risk of cognitive decline and dementia.[16] A meta-analysis review also determined that people who have lower levels of both EPA and DHA as compared with their control group have a higher risk of developing dementia.[17]

A study of over 1,500 healthy adults without dementia found significantly smaller brain volumes and lower scores in tests of visual memory, executive function, and abstract thinking in those with lower DHA in red blood cells.[18] A lab study using fish oil as the source of essential fatty acids showed that it reduced LPS inflammation, reduced amyloid protein production, and had the potential to reduce neuroinflammation in neurodegenerative diseases.[19] Both of these studies underscore how important essential fatty acids are to healthy brain function in general—and specifically in areas that impact on MS symptoms and progression.

Despite a general acceptance that omega-3 fats are essential for good brain health, not all of the clinical trials with Alzheimer's patients have been promising for improving cognitive function; clinical studies involving patients with early stages of mild cognitive impairment or normal cognition do show promising results.[20]

There may be legitimate reasons that some studies with AD patients failed. Some of the causes for failure may be that the daily EFA dosages used were not high enough to be therapeutic, that the treatment duration was not long enough, and that later-stage cognitive decline may not be reversible. Studies that involved patients with moderate to late-stage cognitive loss rarely have positive outcomes, but it's possible that omega-3 fats are effective only when used preventively or in the early stages of cognitive decline.[21]

Research on AD patients with early-stage impairment or normal cognition shows improvements in working memory, immediate verbal memory, and learning skills. More research is needed to better understand how the benefits of omega-3 fats can be optimized to reduce the rate of dementia and neurodegenerative diseases in our aging population.

Other Dietary Intervention Research

In 2014 a more comprehensive review of alternative medicine treatments for MS was published by the American Academy of Neurology, with a broader inclusion criteria.[22] Many of the treatments researched were considered ineffective, based on negative research outcomes or poor research quality. However, some of the reviewed studies were found promising. Only three studies related to omega-3 supplementation in conjunction with a low-fat diet qualified for this review, and the outcome was that it was ineffective in reducing relapse and disability and alleviating symptoms of fatigue. Several cannabis studies were reviewed, and some were found to be somewhat helpful in reducing spasticity and pain. (For more about cannabis and MS treatment, see the "Endocannabinoids" section later in this chapter.)

A large research project conducted under the auspices of St. Vincent's Hospital in Melbourne, Australia, that studied interventions for MS, with the interesting acronym HOLISM (Health Outcomes and Lifestyle Intervention in a Sample of People with Multiple Sclerosis), surveyed over 2,000 people internationally with confirmed disease, and collected data on their level of disability, relapse rates, and daily dietary habits.[23] The data was collected in an online survey, and follow-up occurred over the course of five years. Their results found that a high intake of fruits, vegetables, and healthy fats (omega-3 and -6) was positively associated with a higher quality of life—physically and mentally—and reduced overall disability.

While the reasons remain unclear, the researchers who conducted the study posit that these findings are due to the fact that fruits and vegetables contain polyphenols and carotenoids, which contribute to reduced inflammation, as well as antioxidants, which counteract damaging oxidation pathways typical in MS.

Another study looked at the effects of consuming a healthy low-fat, plant-based diet for one year, as compared with eating an unrestricted diet.[24] To evaluate how the plant-based diet influenced MS signs and symptoms, the research team utilized MRI brain scans and measured relapses, disability, BMI, blood sugar levels, quality-of-life factors, and level of fatigue. The group assigned to the plant-based diet consumed significantly fewer calories in fat. Although this small study did not show significant differences in brain MRI outcomes, relapses, or degree of disability, those consuming a healthy diet showed significant improvements in their levels of fatigue. In conclusion, diet did not change the progression of the illness, but did help with lessening fatigue, which is one of the most debilitating symptoms of MS.

Calorie restriction for treating MS has also been studied. Restricting calories showed some benefit in quality of life when combined with a semi-vegetarian diet based on the Mediterranean diet, including 50 percent carbohydrates, 30 percent protein, low gluten intake, and more fish than meat. Further study needs to be done to confirm these findings, however, because in this study patients self-reported the benefits, as measured by higher quality-of-life scores compared with a control group.[25]

A meta-analysis similar to the Cochrane review on diets for MS was published in 2016, and included a broader range of studies (some of which were mentioned above).[26] In this review of diet and nutrient supplementation studies, authors concluded that dietary factors impact certain parameters, such as fatigue, relapse rate, and disability in MS. They also indicated that diet may play a role in MS development and progression. Based on what they learned from other studies, they recommended a healthy diet low in salt, sugar, and saturated fats. They stated that diets should include an abundance .of fruits and vegetables and avoid processed foods, and that consuming large quantities of meat and dairy has been found to increase the risk of developing MS. This review article also linked obesity in childhood and early adolescence to an increased risk of developing MS, in part because obesity is characterized by higher inflammation. Obesity in MS patients is also linked with increased disability, lower quality of life, increased fatigue, and delayed diagnosis. Given the strong link between MS and obesity, adopting a healthy diet would be especially valuable to young people who want to lower their risk of developing MS.

Types of Diets

Of course, wading through piles of scientific research isn't ordinarily something most people who aren't in the field choose to do; it's far easier to rely on diets that integrate the science into easy-to-follow "prescriptions." But even *that* isn't so easy, because the realm of possibilities is vast, and knowing where to start—or which diet might be most beneficial—isn't automatically intuitive. I know this from personal experience.

Intermittent Fasting

Studies indicate that intermittent fasting (IF)—a pattern of eating in which you spend more time not eating versus eating during a 24-hour period—may improve brain function and protect against cognitive decline. There are several approaches to IF, but the one I personally follow is known as the 16/8 method. In this approach, you restrict the period of eating to 8 hours during the day, and you fast for the 16 hours in between. For a good deal of those 16 hours you'll be asleep, which makes it easier not to eat! Moreover, there is some evidence that avoiding eating at night (rather than caloric restriction itself) is what provides health benefits, because it synchronizes our physiology and metabolism with our natural circadian rhythms. (Note that, as I do, you can use intermittent fasting in tandem with any of the following diets; it's an overall behavior rather than a specific type of eating.)

Ketogenic Diet

Chances are you've heard or read about the ketogenic (keto) diet. It can be a challenging one to follow due its extremely restrictive nature—but it may be worth trying as part of your MS management regimen.

There are many variations on the ketogenic diet, but they all stress a very low intake of carbohydrates, high fat intake, and moderate protein intake. Some keto diets stress dairy as the best source of fat and include eggs. Another version emphasizes supplementing with medium-chain triglycerides as a source of healthy fats; this version allows slightly higher carbohydrate intake.

The human body prefers to use carbohydrates in order to generate the glucose it uses for energy (ATP), but a ketogenic diet instead triggers the body to use organic compounds called *ketones* that result from fat breakdown. Following this diet puts the body into a state of *ketosis*, in which the body releases fatty acids from fat stores. Those fatty acids are converted into ketones in the liver. This process causes the body to become very efficient at burning fat for energy, which is beneficial for weight reduction and reducing blood sugar levels. Ketones can cross the blood-brain barrier and provide a source of fuel for most of the cells of the brain as a substitute for glucose. The benefits increase over time; the longer this low-carb diet is maintained, the more efficiently the brain uses ketones as a source of energy. To achieve a state of ketosis, it is necessary to consume fewer than 50 grams of carbohydrates per day.

The ketogenic diet has long been used as a treatment for epilepsy, especially in situations where standard medications are ineffective.[27] It's not well understood why this works. Some studies have demonstrated that ketone bodies have neuroprotective properties. They may also stimulate new mitochondria production. Ketone bodies increase the levels of glutathione (a compound that protects against cellular damage from free radicals, heavy metals, and other substances) in mitochondria, have antioxidant properties, increase energy production, and help normalize neurologic function. Following a ketogenic diet will increase glutathione levels, but it would be much easier to do so by supplementing with precursors—taking glutathione or precursors of glutathione with N-acetyl cysteine itself. Because of these properties of ketone bodies, a ketogenic diet may be useful in staving off the effects of aging and related neuronal decline. And because it reduces blood sugar levels, a keto diet is an excellent treatment for diabetes.

There is interest in using ketogenic diets for patients with Alzheimer's disease, in part because of its similarities to epilepsy. One clinical trial with AD patients showed that a ketogenic diet that included medium-chain triglycerides (found in coconut oil and dairy products) improved cognitive function in certain types of AD. Ketones also appear to be beneficial in protecting against the toxic effects of beta-amyloid proteins.

In theory a keto diet could prove helpful for MS based on the protective biochemical actions that ketones offer. A keto diet counteracts several of the initial destructive pathways that occur in MS. It reduces oxidation by increasing glutathione levels, supports mitochondrial function, protects against neuron damage, and has anti-inflammatory effects. However, to date, there are no clinical studies that support the use of ketogenic diets in MS. The keto diet can be very hard to follow: It's highly restrictive, for starters, and the changes in eating habits aren't as simple as "eat less bread and pasta," because many healthy fruits and vegetables are high in carbs. I suspect that most patients don't stick to keto or Paleo diets long-term. The trick is to find a diet that is sustainable over many years.

Paleo Diet

Terry Wahls, MD—a physician and medical professor who once suffered from debilitating MS, and is now renowned for her pioneering work on reversing the disease through diet, supplementation, and lifestyle adjustments—has extensively researched the Paleolithic diet. Her modified version of it (included in her protocol for MS patients, known as the Wahls Protocol) is designed to resemble the eating pattern of humans during the Paleolithic period (over 10,000 years ago)—which immediately rules out some of our favorite Western foods, such as pizza, doughnuts, and cookies. Instead, the Paleo diet prescribes fish and lean meats, leafy green vegetables, brightly colored fruits, plant- and animal-derived fats, healthy PUFA oils, and very low carbs. Eggs and gluten are not allowed, because of the high likelihood of allergic responses and inflammation.

The aspect of the Wahls diet that I recommend following is the focus on eating so many vegetables, berries, and grass-fed meat. The diet specifies consuming 9 cups of fruits and vegetables daily: 3 cups of greens, 3 cups of darkly pigmented vegetables, and 3 cups of high-sulfur vegetables.

Cabbage-family vegetables—such as broccoli, cabbage, and cauliflower—and garlic and onions are rich in sulfur and therefore highly recommended because of their role in supporting glutathione production and detoxification. High intake of leafy green vegetables, such as kale, spinach, and Swiss chard, offers high doses of vitamin K_2, which is a nutritional cofactor in producing myelin. Dark-pigmented fruits and vegetables, such as eggplant and berries, offer high levels of polyphenols for neuroprotection and antioxidant activity. They are also excellent for reducing inflammation. Meats should be grass-fed; organ meats and wild fish are also acceptable.

Dr. Wahls has published two small clinical studies to evaluate the benefits of the Wahls Protocol—which, besides the modified Paleo diet, incorporates supplements and lifestyle activities such as massage, neuromuscular electrical stimulation, acupuncture, and meditation.[28] Both studies showed that the MS patients reported progressive improvement in their fatigue, mood, and cognitive symptoms over the course of the one-year trial. These are important indicators that strongly influence the quality of life for MS patients.

The Paleo diet has some similarities to the ketogenic diet, but it is much less restrictive and easier to manage in the long term. It allows for greater flexibility in food choices—especially considering it doesn't eliminate whole-food carbs found in many fruits and vegetables, as the keto diet does—and it doesn't require complicated daily calculations of macronutrients to ensure the "correct" ratio. Dr. Wahls finds the ketogenic diet difficult to sustain and has expressed concern about potential health problems for those who follow it over the long term; it may put patients at greater risk for nutritional deficiencies, hormone interference, and microbiome disruption. I personally think that any diet that is so restrictive, and that causes any nutrient deficiencies, is problematic.

Swank Diet

One of the best-known dietary treatments for MS, the Swank diet, attempts to control disease progression through very low intake of saturated fat.[29] The Swank diet limits fats to 50 grams per day. No more than 20 grams of the total can be saturated fat. The diet allows for two servings per day of low-fat dairy products and four servings per day of grains, including bread and pasta. It also allows eggs.

Helminth Therapy

Population studies have shown that autoimmune conditions like MS occur much less frequently in people who are infected with parasitic worms known as *helminths*. The theory is that parasitic helminths evolved over several millennia in consort with the immune systems of mammals. To maximize their chances of survival, the helminths became very adept at down-modulating the immune response of their host so that the host immune system would not be activated to attack the helminths. This modulation of the host's immunity may have had the (side) effect of protecting the host from excessive inflammatory and autoimmune reactivity. This observation has been corroborated in animal models of autoimmunity; mice infected with helminth parasites are protected from the progression of MS. Many other parasites also appear to have this protective effect against MS in experimental models.

These findings have sparked interest in exploring the therapeutic application of helminth infections in patients with autoimmune conditions. A few studies of MS have looked at using the eggs of the helminth parasite *Trichuris suis*, and the larvae of *Necator americanus*. These studies have been small and of short duration and have mainly looked at safety. A study of five MS patients using *Trichuris suis* reported a decrease in the development of new CNS lesions during and up to two months following treatment, as well as increased blood levels of two anti-inflammatory cytokines. Another study of 12 MS patients that used a variety of helminths showed they had fewer relapses and MRI changes when compared with MS patients who were not infected. So far, no adverse events have been reported.

As an alternative to using live helminth infections, research is ongoing to identify chemicals derived from helminth parasites that can modulate the immune system and potentially mimic the protective effects of parasitic infection. Even though administering helminthic infections has had positive results in mouse models of MS and early preclinical studies, if you want to explore helminthic therapy using live parasites or ova (eggs), I strongly recommend that you do so only under knowledgeable medical supervision or as part of a controlled clinical study.

The diet became popularized because of positive results of a clinical trial begun in the early 1950s by Dr. Roy Swank. Results of the study showed that strictly following the Swank dietary guidelines resulted in reduced relapse rates, less disability, and better overall survival over a 50-year follow-up. The study had shortcomings, though: It lacked a control group to compare outcomes against; there was a high dropout rate among study participants; and, because MRI technology hadn't yet been developed, there was no way to image participants' brains before and after the study to qualitatively determine what changes may have occurred.

When I was diagnosed with MS, I followed the Swank diet religiously for six months, and my symptoms—as well as my lesions detected via MRI—significantly *worsened*. I question the approach of this diet from a metabolic perspective. The brain is made up of fat, and it seems counterintuitive to remove a compound that is essential to neurological development and function. It is important to include organic high-quality fat in the diet. (I'll note here that we do have to be careful to avoid ingesting foods containing fats that have been extracted with toxic solvents, or oxidized, or heated.)

Hormone production also relies on adequate cholesterol (which the body generates from fat), and we know that hormone balance plays a role in MS progression. It's still not well understood how a severely low-fat diet such as the Swank diet would be beneficial in a neurodegenerative disease. To better understand this question, Dr. Wahls is collaborating with the National Multiple Sclerosis Society to conduct a clinical trial, funded by the National Institutes of Health, comparing the effectiveness of the Paleo diet versus the Swank diet on reducing fatigue in patients with MS.[30] This study is in progress at the time of this writing.

Mediterranean Diet

The Mediterranean diet is more liberal than the Paleo, as it includes some foods that are eliminated or restricted in the Paleo counterpart. The Mediterranean diet includes olive oil, whole grains, vegetables, fish, legumes, and some dairy. It does not specify ratios of each food category, but generally fruits, vegetables, legumes, nuts, and whole grains dominate the diet. Red meat is only rarely eaten, and sugar and processed foods are avoided entirely.

A scientific review of the Mediterranean diet found it counteracts inflammation and neurodegenerative diseases. In a published paper, the reviewers suggest that inflammation accelerates as we age, thus dubbing it "inflammaging."[31] Aging increases the risk of developing inflammation-related chronic diseases such as diabetes, arthritis, and neurodegenerative issues. The abundance of antioxidants and phenols provided by the Mediterranean diet has been found to reduce inflammation. Epidemiologic studies have shown that people who consistently consume a Mediterranean diet have a lower risk of developing chronic illnesses and neurodegenerative diseases. However, as mentioned earlier in the book, gluten and some other grains arguably could (and even should) be avoided due to their potential inflammatory and allergic properties.

I tried many kinds of diets before settling mostly on the Mediterranean diet, weaving in some aspects of the Paleo diet, such as limiting sugars and wheat. My advice? Don't be intimidated; do your own research on diets, decide which seem most appealing and manageable to you, and give them a try—one at a time, of course, because you don't want to muddy the results. If you're methodical and record any changes (both positive and negative) you experience while following a particular diet, you can dial in your eating in a way that helps you feel the best that you can.

Supplements and Drugs

Supplements and herbs aren't all subject to the same large-scale clinical trials that pharmaceuticals are; and those trials are what many physicians rely upon as the green light for them to prescribe. They're trained not to be comfortable with the idea of prescribing ingredients that have not gone through large clinical review trials.

That said, the supplements I discuss in this chapter *have* been widely studied. I've both recommended them to my patients in the past and used them myself, often to great benefit. As with diet, some may work better for you than others; I've provided what I hope to be useful information about their effects so you can make an informed decision about which to try.

I also recommend some pharmaceuticals that are showing promise in the treatment of MS, based on their efficacy in other conditions. In the case of supplements, please do consult a health care practitioner who is knowledgeable about restorative medicine *before* adding them to your medicine chest. It's always a good idea for everyone to be on the same page when it comes to your overall treatment plan! Discussing supplements and asking for guidance with conventional physicians is usually not fruitful, at least in my experience.

Cordyceps sinensis

Cordyceps—also called dong chong xia cao, or "winter-worm summer-plant"— is a fungus that parasitizes small caterpillars and beetles found in higher altitudes of the Tibetan plateau. Due to its relative rarity, *Cordyceps* has been revered as an energy, immune, and longevity tonic used mainly by the elite. It has long been established as an important traditional medicine with numerous uses in China, Tibet, Korea, and Japan. It has been used to treat conditions ranging from infections, cancer, and chronic inflammatory diseases to heart disease, neurological disease, and brain disorders, including memory loss and senility. For all of these traditional indications, *Cordyceps* is often classified as an adaptogen.

Rosmarinic acid

Rosmarinic acid is an extract of the rosemary plant. It supports healthy immune system and thyroid function and normal histamine production. *Note:* If rosmarinic acid upsets your stomach, as it can mine, you can take an herb called marshmallow root to soothe the irritation.

On its own, rosmarinic acid has been shown to stimulate myelin growth in the corpus callosum and increase the production of oligodendrocytes in animal studies. It also has been shown to be neuroprotective against the various modes of neuronal cell death.

Glutathione

This antioxidant has increasingly been linked to cognitive function, especially in older adults.[32] Studies are under way to learn the specific reasons for this effect, and why people with higher levels of glutathione in their blood enjoy better cognitive function than those with normal or low levels. Generally speaking, however, glutathione reduces oxidative stress in the brain by helping cells to repair themselves—which also supports and maintains connections among neurons.

Vitamin D₃

It's not surprising that the highest rates of multiple sclerosis occur in parts of the world where sunshine is limited—low vitamin D level is closely correlated to autoimmune dysfunction. Researchers have definitively linked low vitamin D levels to a variety of neurological and cognitive impairments. Here in North America, the highest rates of MS occur in Canada, followed by Vermont. People who were born and raised in Texas are among the least likely to develop MS. And among people who live on or near the equator, almost no one has, or will develop, multiple sclerosis.

I had always freely prescribed vitamin D to my patients who suffer from autoimmune diseases. Once I learned of my own diagnosis, I began taking it myself.

When prescribing, I generally start at 2,000 IU daily, taken indefinitely. When I do this, my patients often say, "That's a *lot* of vitamin D!" It is—and that's by design. The sooner you can elevate your vitamin D levels and keep them high, the better chance of having a healthy immune response.

Fish Oils

Have you ever heard the expression that "fish is food for your brain"? It's true. Researchers have discovered a direct link between omega-3 oils, found predominantly in fatty fish like tuna and salmon, and cognitive health. People with low plasma levels of omega-3s such as DHA and EPA are at greater risk for visual impediments, disturbances in learning, decline in overall cognitive health, and certain kinds of dementia, including Alzheimer's.

Eating more fish certainly helps. I try to take 2 teaspoons of cod liver oil a day. During exacerbations, I might double the dosage.

As an added bonus, fish oil can help decrease inflammation during an active MS attack. I recommend 1 teaspoon of fish oil five times per day in this situation. I've done this, and found it useful. Something to consider!

Fumarate

Dimethyl fumarate (DMF) is derived from fumaric acid and is a standard treatment for psoriasis, a condition that, like MS, has origins in autoimmunity.

The precise mechanism of action for fumarate is not well understood, but it appears to be multifactorial. It has an anti-inflammatory action that positively affects the immune system in order to reduce the autoimmune reaction. It also acts on macrophages, microglia, and neurons as an antioxidant and neuroprotectant.[33] Lab studies suggest that the potent antioxidant activity is due to fumaric acid's effect on glutathione levels. Glutathione is considered a master antioxidant; it is synthesized in the body, is oxidized (used up), and then recycled in the liver to be used again. Fumaric acid appears to have the ability to enhance glutathione levels, even when endogenous production is low, by upregulating glutathione recycling via supporting one of the enzymes responsible for the process.[34]

Early clinical trials of DMF on MS patients were small, but showed promise in terms of efficacy and safety. Later, large multicenter trials were initiated. A two-year, multicenter study called the Comparator and an Oral Fumarate in Relapsing-Remitting Multiple Sclerosis (CONFIRM) trial included over 1,400 patients who took one of two dosage options of DMF, a placebo, or another drug called glatiramer acetate (GA) over the two-year trial. The higher dose of DMF caused a 51 percent reduction in relapse rate, and the lower dose led to 44 percent reduction, both as compared with placebo. The DMF results were more impressive than the GA medication, which reduced relapse by just 29 percent over placebo. DMF also beat out GA in terms of reducing the number of new or enlarging lesions as determined by an MRI scan (scans were performed on only a subset of patients). The reduction in relapses was shown to have had a positive effect on the overall quality of life for the patients. Subsequent clinical trials affirmed the results of the CON-FIRM trial. Researchers learned that initiating treatment in the early stages of MS leads to a much better outcome, especially if initiated before neuronal damage starts.

Fumaric acid esters are also being investigated for their potential role in recovery from traumatic brain injury, which is known to potentially lead to neurodegeneration over time. Animal studies show that it may be neuropro-tective via anti-inflammatory activity.[35]

DMF is available as a prescription drug with the trade name Tecfidera. (I have tried it, but it was not effective for me.) Studies have shown that DMF is very safe, with only mild side effects, such as gastrointestinal complaints and temporary skin flushing. GI symptoms include mild to moderate diarrhea, nausea, vomiting, and abdominal pain and discomfort, and these side effects tend to diminish over time. There are no known drug interactions, and so far Tecfidera seems safe to use during pregnancy.

Fumaric acid is also available in the form of a dietary supplement, but GI absorption may be too limited for it to be effective. Shepherd's purse and a few other herbs are known to naturally contain the sour-tasting compound fumaric acid. Some of the plant sources have been used in traditional herbal medicine for skin conditions, but to date there is no research that demon-strates their efficacy in treating MS.

Resveratrol

Resveratrol is a polyphenol derived from grapes and red wine. It is the compound responsible for giving wine its cardioprotective effects, a potent antioxidant that also offers neuroprotection through reducing inflamma-tion. Cell studies show that resveratrol reduces amyloid protein production and protects microglial nerve cells from damage.[36] Animal studies suggest that resveratrol may prevent beta-amyloid plaque development and reduce neuroinflammation.[37] Several clinical trials demonstrate that resveratrol enhances brain function by causing vasorelaxation and improving blood flow to the brain.

Research indicates that resveratrol has the potential to benefit most neurodegenerative diseases.[38] It can reduce oxidative stress in Parkinson's disease that is produced by the accumulation of Lewy bodies. In Huntington's disease it may be beneficial through reducing oxidation caused by mitochondrial dysfunctions and huntingtin protein accumulation. (Huntingtin protein is found throughout the body, but its highest concentrations are in the brain, where it exists in neurons and glial cells.)[39] In Alzheimer's disease it may reduce the oxidative stress caused by amyloid-beta proteins. And in MS resveratrol can be neuroprotective against glutamate neurotoxicity.[40]

One animal study has found that resveratrol could possibly exacerbate autoimmune demyelination.[41] However, a later animal study found that resveratrol contributed to remyelination. More research is needed to better understand how resveratrol might benefit patients with MS. In the meanwhile, I take resveratrol in the form of drinking a glass of red wine with dinner.

Curcumin

The bright gold Indian culinary spice called turmeric (*Curcuma longa*) offers great promise for neuroprotection. It contains the polyphenolic compound curcumin, which has recently become one of the most popular supplements in the United States—and with good reason. Curcumin is one of the most extensively researched plant compounds, in part because it has such broad health benefits. Curcumin is known to support the body's systemic anti-inflammatory response, and historically it has been used for inflammatory conditions such as arthritis.[42] Because it has the ability to cross the blood-brain barrier, curcumin is a very effective neuroprotectant. Curcumin reduces inflammation and oxidation and shows promise for reducing amyloid-beta production and existing plaque. It has been shown to reduce amyloid-beta-induced cognitive decline and reduce microglia activity to slow or prevent neurodegeneration. Human and animal studies show that curcumin improves cognitive function and memory impairment, possibly via its antioxidant activity and or support for new neuronal development. Animal studies show that curcumin increases the production of neuronal cells and increases the growth of neuron extensions in the areas of the brain related to memory. Therefore, long-term consumption should enhance memory. Many studies, in fact, have shown that curcumin can improve cognition overall.

For these reasons, curcumin has been studied as a preventive agent against the progression of Parkinson's and Alzheimer's diseases.[43] It also looks promising as a protector against neuroinflammation, in part because it is absorbed through the blood-brain barrier and remains active in the brain. Curcumin appears to moderate inflammation through a variety of mechanisms including targeting oxidative stress and mitochondrial dysfunction, both of which play a direct role in neurodegenerative processes.

Although much of our understanding about the effects of curcumin on neurodegeneration come from cell and animal studies, a few clinical trials have been conducted, and the outcomes are variable.[44] A review of five clinical trials on curcumin and cognitive decline determined that only two of the five had positive outcomes, and both involved healthy participants without diagnosed neurodegenerative diseases. The studies used different brands and forms of curcumin, and the dosages ranged from 400 mg to 4 grams per day. Interestingly, the lower doses had the more positive outcomes and did not cause side effects, in comparison with the high-dose studies, which had reports of GI distress. The two positive studies showed improvements in memory with either short- or long-term consumption of curcumin. The other three studies did not show significant improvements in cognitive function, although two of the three negative trials involved patients with Alzheimer's disease diagnoses. As mentioned previously, reversing chronic neurodegeneration is challenging and typically has a low success rate. In the negative study with healthy participants, the placebo group did not experience cognitive decline, so there was no apparent difference between the treatment and placebo group at the end of the study.

Curcumin bioavailability is a much-debated topic by supplement companies in order to market it. However, in reality, it's not all that complicated. Taking curcumin or its extracts mixed with a fat, or with the essential oils of turmeric, is helpful with absorption.[45] Curcumin has low water solubility, and it is metabolized to other compounds once absorbed, which consequently makes it difficult to detect in the blood. On the positive side, because the compound is more fat-soluble than water-soluble, it is absorbed through the blood-brain barrier and can be detected as being active in the brain. I take curcumin in the form of "golden milk," a hot or cold beverage with coconut milk and honey. I also take daily capsules of curcumin extracts mixed with the essential oils. This is a product I designed called Enfla-Mend.

Holy Basil

Holy basil (*Ocimum tenuiflorum*) is another herb that has been used medicinally for thousands of years and is now being investigated for its possible benefit in neurodegenerative disorders. Most of the studies so far have used animal or in vitro (test tube) models, but the findings suggest holy basil may have neuroprotective actions. One study found that an ethanol extract of *O. tenuiflorum* improved cognitive function in younger rats by maintaining the activity of a chemical known as choline acetyltransferase (ChAT). ChAT promotes the production of acetylcholine, a neurotransmitter that is critical in humans for cognition, learning, memory, and muscle control. This study is significant because, for reasons that are poorly understood, dementia can sometimes affect young and middle-aged people; the younger animal model used in this experiment could indicate a potential benefit for holy basil in those populations.

In another study, an ethanol extract of *Ocimum tenuiflorum* was applied to human cells in an in vitro model of neurodegenerative disease. In this study holy basil extract prevented nerve cell death and maintained ChAT levels for the continued production of acetylcholine.

I take holy basil as a hot tea or in capsule form. Despite being from Asia, it grows great here in Vermont. My friend grows it very well on his farm called Zack Woods. It is available online as well.

Ashwagandha

Ashwagandha (*Withania somnifera*) is another traditional herbal medicine that has undergone extensive scientific study. Results indicate that ashwagandha may prove to be an ally in alleviating neuroinflammation. Ashwagandha is an adaptogenic herb, which means it enhances the body's ability to respond to internal and external stressors in a healthy way by modulating the activity of the hypothalamic-pituitary-adrenal (HPA) axis. When the HPA axis is chronically activated because of prolonged exposure to stress (a common problem in our modern lifestyle), it can result in sustained high levels or dysregulated levels of the stress hormone cortisol. Studies show that chronically high levels of cortisol may play a role in cognitive and memory impairment. In addition to its modulation of the HPA axis, ashwagandha may also exert its influence through other biochemical mechanisms. An in vitro study that looked at human nerve cells showed that ashwagandha was protective against the formation of beta-amyloid protein plaques. In a study with rats, ashwagandha and withanolide A (one of ashwagandha's major bioactive ingredients) were shown to almost completely reverse impairments in spatial memory. In these examples it is possible that ashwagandha promoted antioxidant activity and mitigated oxidative stress.

Like golden milk with turmeric, I also enjoy a beverage made from mixing ashwagandha with coconut milk and honey. The traditional East Indian recipe is made with cow's milk.

Endocannabinoids / CBD products

Many states are legalizing medical cannabis, and interest in the role of the endocannabinoid system in the body is increasing. Until recently, the role of this system was not taught in medical schools, and therefore it has never been a focus for medical treatments. What exactly is it? The endogenous endocannabinoid system intersects with various other systems of the body, aiding in communication and coordination for different cell types. The primary purpose of the endocannabinoid system seems to be establishing balance throughout the body. Various types of cannabinoid receptors are found throughout the body and influence many different systems. From the perspective of neurodegenerative disease, the most interesting aspect is that cannabinoids are naturally present in our bodies, and the cannabinoids that are extracted from cannabis plants have been shown to help regulate the function of both the immune system and the nervous system. In the nervous system, cannabinoids moderate nerve synapses and neurotransmitter release.

In the immune system, cannabinoids influence inflammatory responses by inhibiting certain immune cells, including the microglia cells, which have cannabinoid receptors. This can reduce chronic inflammation and ultimately protect the neurons.[46]

Activation of certain endocannabinoid receptors has been shown to delay progression of neurodegeneration. Animal studies show that cannabinoid compounds reduce inflammation in the nervous system and improve neurological symptoms. And many of the neuroinflammatory processes involved in ALS have been shown to be tempered by activating endocannabinoid receptors.

Another way that endocannabinoids can be both neuroprotective and anti-inflammatory is by limiting excitatory factors such as glutamate. Glutamate is an amino acid that can overexcite the nervous system and increase oxidative stress. An example of this is sensitivity to MSG (monosodium glutamate) that leads to a physical reaction such as a migraine. In the case of MS, excitatory glutamate acts to accelerate the disease progression, but the endocannabinoid system may potentially play a role in tempering that.

Not all research on cannabinoids has been positive. So far, studies using synthetic cannabinoids to treat MS have shown some effectiveness in treating pain or spasticity in MS, with mixed results for treating other related symptoms.

I have tried CBD, but have not felt any benefit from it. I wonder whether the enthusiasm about CBD is being driven by equity firms who have invested in marketing CBD products. Although I am somewhat skeptical about CBD, others have told me that it has helped them.

Improving Oxygen Supply

The brain needs oxygen. High levels of oxygen in the CNS actually inhibit demyelination in animal studies. Oxygen is transported by the blood throughout the body, where it stimulates the release of growth factors and stem cells to promote healing. Among the many simple activities and lifestyle adjustments that promote oxygen supply to the brain are physical exercise, yoga, breathing techniques (such as alternate nostril breathing), restorative sleep, and avoiding toxins like cigarettes and alcohol. Hyperbaric oxygen therapy, the use of oxygen concentrators, and venous angioplasty are three technical interventions that significantly improve oxygenation.

Hyperbaric Oxygen

I have not seen any benefit from hyperbaric oxygen therapy myself. Nonetheless, some MS patients have. Hyperbaric oxygen therapy (HBOT) entails sitting in a hyperbaric oxygen chamber in which air pressure is increased, usually to three times higher than normal air pressure. This allows the lungs to process more oxygen than would be possible at normal air pressure using pure (100 percent) oxygen. Mixed results have been reported in HBOT studies, but this may be due in part to a lack of consistency in the standards for HBOT. Scientific evidence for using HBOT to successfully treat autoimmune disorders and reduce neuroinflammation is considered insufficient. However, people with MS have been self-managing their symptoms with HBOT for decades and have reported positive effects, especially with bladder control. HBOT has also been shown to stabilize symptoms of MS, slow its progression, and potentially reverse cognitive issues during the period of time that patients actively engage in the therapy. Benefits diminish over time as the therapy is discontinued,

HBOT Information for Practitioners

Professor Philip James, an expert in the use of hyperbaric oxygen therapy, recommends the following therapeutic protocol:

- Plan for a minimum of 20 sessions over a period of four to six weeks to begin with, and then ideally 1 per week.
- Start with an oxygen pressure at 1.5 atm for five sessions.
- If no noticeable benefit occurs, then increase to 1.75 atm for five sessions.
- If no noticeable benefit is yet evident, then increase to 2.0 atm for the remainder of the sessions, but do not expose patients to pressures above 2 atm. Above 2 atm, the dose-response curve is very erratic and the secondary vasoconstriction may outweigh the benefit of the increased oxygen.

however. For best results, therefore, use HBOT on a weekly basis at least. This is a sensible recommendation, and not an onerous one: By comparison, most other drug and injection therapies for MS are required on a daily basis.

Oxygen Concentrators

An oxygen concentrator is an electronic device that concentrates oxygen by taking in ambient air and filtering out nitrogen. It delivers purified oxygen via a mask or nasal cannula. It is recommended that you find a machine that provides a flow rate of 12 liters per minute. This will allow you to use it for exercise with oxygen therapy (EWOT), which is exactly what the term suggests: inhaling concentrated oxygen while you're exercising. Ideally, you'll EWOT during interval training three times a week. An oxygen concentrator is noisy, but you can use one while sleeping by putting the machine in a separate room from your bedroom. A small tube extends from the machine into your bedroom to transport the purified oxygen and release it inside the pillowcase of your pillow, increasing ambient oxygen near your nose and mouth throughout the night, which can improve your oxygen saturation levels.

I try to keep my oxygen levels high by deep breathing from my diaphragm, a technique I have learned in yoga classes. It is easy to measure your oxygen levels at home with a pulse oximeter—a very affordable device that can be bought online or at a pharmacy without a prescription. It's a great way to measure how your breathing impacts your oxygen levels.

Venous Angioplasty

A researcher in Italy, Dr. Paolo Zamboni, has proposed that chronic cerebrospinal venous insufficiency (CCSVI) may contribute to the CNS damage seen in MS. CCSVI is an abnormality in the way blood drains from the brain and spinal cord. The treatment Dr. Zamboni offered for CCSVI is angioplasty, a procedure in which blocked or narrowed veins are opened by inflating a small balloon in them or inserting a stent to improve blood flow and blood drainage from the brain. In the case of MS patients, the veins operated on would usually be both internal jugular veins, the azygos vein, and the left renal vein. Research showing a link between vein abnormalities and MS has been mixed. The FDA has also issued a statement of concern about the safety and effectiveness of venous angioplasty. However, it may be a promising emerging therapy and appears to have helped many MS patients.

CHAPTER 6

Reinsulating the Wires

Earlier in the book I described myelin as an insulating sheath that protects axons and speeds the rate at which nerve impulses travel along the central nervous system. I also talked about the significance of demyelination and its relationship to neurodegenerative diseases like MS. *Remyelination*, then, is a potentially promising way to slow, halt, or even reverse disease progression. Returning to my original metaphor, remyelination is like reinsulating an electrical wire—restoring the outer coating that protects the integrity of nerve signals.

The exciting news is that the brain does demonstrate some capacity to repair itself, and neurotrophins such as nerve growth factor (NGF) could play a key role. Previously, in chapter 3, I discussed the relationship between high levels of NGF and neuroinflammation; and in chapter 5 I briefly touched on the idea that NGF might positively impact neuroplasticity and the ability to regenerate myelin. It may also help with *adaptive plasticity*, the brain's natural capacity to compensate for nerve-damaging events by producing neurotrophic factors such as NGF. Other neurotrophic factors counteract oxidation and mitochondrial dysfunction. Researchers are still working to understand the complexities of NGF, and some interesting studies have come out that are relevant for MS patients. Also, because of the exciting potential that neurotrophic treatments could offer, much recent drug research has focused on their development.

(There are other promising treatments on the horizon, too. Two pioneering approaches include stem cell therapy and the use of neuropeptides.)

What does all of this mean? That we can take steps now, such as using specific supplements and other therapies, to decrease the intensity and frequency of MS attacks that lead to demyelination. We can also help support the body's ability to repair and remyelinate.

Several supplements, such as PQQ (see below), work to increase NGF levels in the body. Others, also covered below, don't affect NGF but can help to reduce neuroinflammation and support acetylcholine, which helps with memory and learning.

Nerve Growth Factor

People with MS, Alzheimer's disease, and Parkinson's disease generally have low levels of nerve growth factor. NGF is one of a group of proteins called neurotrophins that nurture the development of new neurons and repair and regenerate damaged neurons. (Neurotrophins, in turn, are one of three families that together form a class of growth factors called neurotrophic factors.) NGF controls the critical function of repairing the myelin sheath. NGF also has a wide variety of other actions, including protecting pancreatic cells and balancing immune and hormone activity. It may also help repair the heart after a heart attack by rebuilding damaged blood vessels. Given how many systems rely on NGF, you'd think that having high levels of it would protect against neurodegenerative disease, right? Unfortunately, it's not that simple. In fact, harking back to the concept of balance, too much of a good thing may be harmful.

Scientists acknowledge there is still much to learn about NGF because its role in the body is so complicated. For example, under certain conditions that are not fully understood, white blood cells known as mast cells secrete NGF as part of their inflammatory response during allergic reactions. Mast cells appear in the bloodstream in high numbers in people with certain autoimmune conditions. In addition, in certain autoimmune conditions such as rheumatoid arthritis, high levels of NGF are linked to a higher sensitivity to pain. (Incidentally, this has led pharmaceutical companies to develop drugs that block or reduce levels of NGF as a means of reducing pain.[1]) People with MS who experience high levels of pain and inflammation often have abnormally high levels of NGF in their spinal fluid.[2] However, that can also be the case in people with MS who are *not* experiencing pain. High levels of mast cells can also be found in plaques in the brains of MS patients.[3]

My Personal Prescription for Encouraging Remyelination

In order to most effectively manage MS, I recommend a combination of anti-inflammatory, neuroregenerative, and neuroprotective strategies. I covered the first in chapter 5; here are my recommended, and scientifically researched, approaches for the second—both in the long run and following an acute flare. (I will discuss the third in chapter 8.) You'll notice that some natural medicines appear in more than one category, which is a testament to their potentially wide-ranging beneficial effects.

Do eat (and drink):
• Plenty of berries

Choose these herbs and supplements:
• Lion's mane mushroom
• PQQ
• Rosmarinic acid from rosemary
• Curcumin or turmeric essential oils (turmerones) from turmeric
• Quercetin
• Biotin
• Iodine
• Thyroid hormones

Injections:
• Peptide therapy such as thymosin beta-4

Despite the fact that high levels of NGF are linked to inflammation and autoimmunity, its role in promoting remyelination could mean that it is a net positive for healing neurological damage related to MS. In fact, research has shown that NGF can repair myelin and protect the brain. Rather than labeling NGF as good or bad, a better way to think about it may simply be in terms of balance. The high NGF levels seen in MS may be a *response* to tissue damage rather than the *cause* of it. Most likely, balanced levels of NGF are healthy and beneficial, and levels that are either too low or too high are detrimental. Although scientists don't have complete understanding yet, it is clear that NGF has a positive impact on the nervous system under the right conditions and at the appropriate level. In my opinion, it is usually beneficial to enhance NGF as part of a comprehensive MS treatment plan.

Increasing NGF and Promoting Remyelination

Because MS is a disease characterized by damage to the myelin sheath, remyelination can help to slow progression and reduce symptoms. Increasing levels of NGF in the body may hold potential as a way to promote remyelination. As of this writing, no pharmaceutical drugs are known to increase NGF. However, two classes of natural compounds, one found in a plant and the other derived from a mushroom, have been shown to promote the production of NGF in animal models. These compounds are *turmerones*, which are found in turmeric, and *diterpene derivatives* from the lion's mane mushroom. In addition, the flavonoid *quercetin* has been shown to improve myelination, potentially through a different mechanism than NGF production. And vitamin B_{12} is a nutrient required for myelin synthesis.

Turmerone

Along with curcumin, turmerone is a major bioactive constituent of turmeric. Turmerone has anti-inflammatory effects, particularly against microglia. In addition, turmerone has been shown to promote the production of neural stem cells, which have the capacity to generate neurons and repair nerve damage, as discussed later in this chapter.

Lion's Mane

This medicinal mushroom (*Hericium erinaceus*), which is also known as sheep's head, gets its name from its resemblance to these animals. If you can imagine a large mushroom with long flowing white "hair," that is what lion's mane looks like. Lion's mane contains many bioactive compounds, in particular hericenones and erinacines, that potentially have neuroregenerative and neuroprotective effects. Research indicates that these compounds help reduce amyloid-beta plaque deposition and help reduce neuropathic pain. One of the benefits of the compounds is that they can cross the blood-brain barrier, making them directly available to act on the central nervous system.

Lion's mane has also been reported to promote the production of NGF in nerve cells and to protect nerve cells against damage from neuroinflammation caused by oxidative stress. Neurotrophic factors such as those found in lion's mane are particularly important for maintaining the structure of neurons that produce the neurotransmitter acetylcholine.

Lab studies show that lion's mane extract enhances myelination and improves nerve growth after brain injury. Lion's mane is also protective to nerves when exposed to the toxins that induce Parkinson's disease. Animal studies show that lion's mane prevents memory impairment and reduces amyloid-beta plaque.[4]

Two small clinical trials have been conducted on lion's mane. In one, adults with mild cognitive impairment took lion's mane, in the form of a 250 mg tablet comprising 96 percent dry powder, three times daily for 16 weeks, and were shown to have significant improvement in cognitive function. Within a month of discontinuing the mushroom supplement, subjects' cognitive scores declined. In a second study, postmenopausal women consumed 2 grams of lion's mane per day for four weeks. They experienced a reduction of anxiety and depression as compared with a similar group who did not take the lion's mane.[5]

Depending on potency, the therapeutic dose is up to 5 grams of lion's mane per day. Look for supplements that use the fruiting body rather than mycelium, which does not contain the active compounds. Be aware that most lion's mane supplements available in stores are primarily not the mushroom but the mycelium hairs. According to research (which I helped conduct), the mycelium contains no traceable active constituents. Be sure you are buying products containing the whole mushroom. Fortunately I live in Vermont, where we have several organic mushroom growers who cultivate lion's mane. I cook with it in soups and stir-fries. The best-tasting lion's mane, hands-down, is picked fresh in the woods (but be sure you know how to precisely identify any wild mushroom before consuming it). Lion's mane grows in the early fall in Vermont and is delicious! In the past I have taken it in the form of capsules, but stopped once I was able to eat it fresh.

Lion's mane seems to be very safe and without interactions. However, some individuals may find they are sensitive or allergic to lion's mane.

Quercetin

Quercetin is a flavonoid, which is a type of natural pigment found in many plants and foods, including berries, apples, grapes, cherries, red wine, onions, and green tea. It is a powerful antioxidant, and studies in humans suggest that it may be protective against neurodegenerative disorders. In addition, in some animal models of MS, quercetin prevented demyelination and sped up remyelination of damaged neurons. Quercetin has also been studied for its effects on perinatal cerebral hypoxia/ischemia (PHI)—a condition seen in newborns who suffer from a lack of oxygen to the brain. One of the dangers of PHI is that brain cells do not undergo myelination. In an animal model of cerebral hypoxia/ischemia, quercetin was shown to increase the number of cells that produce oligodendrocytes, which are required for myelination to occur. Quercetin was also shown to protect oligodendrocytes once they formed. Not only did quercetin improve myelination in this animal model, but the cognitive performance of the animals was also shown to improve as a consequence. Quercetin may also have neuroprotective effects by supporting the acetylcholine neurotransmitter system.

PQQ

Pyrroloquinoline quinone (PQQ) is a neuroprotective nutrient found in a variety of vegetables, such as spinach and green peppers, and in kiwifruit, tofu, green tea, and human milk. It can also be taken as a supplement. PQQ helps heal the brain and encourages the growth of new nerve cells. It supports the production of new mitochondria, enhances ATP production, and counteracts oxidative damage.[6] One study demonstrated that mitochondrial function can be enhanced by taking just 13 mg of PQQ daily. In a healthy diet that includes lots of vegetables, you can consume up to 1 mg a day. In another study, people took 20 mg of PQQ daily, resulting in a decrease of the inflammatory marker C-reactive protein.[7]

PQQ also stimulates NGF in brain cells, as demonstrated in lab studies. In theory, increasing NGF helps with nerve growth and repair and improves neuroplasticity to improve memory and learning.[8] Studies with older animals show that PQQ helps increase the rate of learning new information and improves memory, via increased production of NGF.

PQQ also helps reduce neuroinflammation by limiting pro-inflammatory cytokines, as shown in animal research on traumatic brain injury.[9] PQQ may help reduce excitotoxicity, a process that damages, and can even kill, neurons when the receptors for glutamate overactivate. One animal study showed that PQQ helped counteract the neurotoxic effects of glutamate on brain cells and significantly reduced the degree of damage from oxidation. PQQ also helps the body use coenzyme Q10 (CoQ10) and vitamin D_3 more efficiently. This is significant because CoQ10 has powerful antioxidant and anti-inflammatory actions, and low levels of vitamin D have been linked to autoimmunity and to neurological and cognitive impairments.

Vitamin B_{12}

Vitamin B_{12}, also known as cobalamin, is necessary for the proper formation of myelin. In fact, in the absence of sufficient B_{12}, myelin will be defective. Symptoms of B_{12} deficiency include numbness and tingling in the hands and feet; fatigue; balance problems; and memory issues. (Notice that all of these symptoms may also be experienced by people with MS.) Although there isn't any evidence linking B_{12} supplementation with improvement in MS symptoms, it's worth considering using it, given its importance as a cofactor for myelin production. Also of interest: Because vitamin B_{12} improves fatigue, it potentially can help alleviate this common and troublesome symptom of MS.

Biotin

Biotin is a B-complex vitamin found in a wide array of foods including egg yolks, organ meats, cheese, leafy green vegetables, sweet potato, nuts, seeds, and raw cauliflower. It is considered an essential vitamin, which means that it must be obtained from dietary sources; the human body cannot make its own biotin. Biotin is required for many crucial metabolic processes, including fatty acid synthesis (and as previously explained, fatty acids are necessary for myelin production) and the conversion of nutrients to energy that the body can use to ensure sufficient oxygenation of tissues. Biotin is one of the most researched natural substances for possible benefits for humans with MS because of its potential to increase energy production in damaged nerves and to repair demyelination.[10] There is no recommended dietary allowance (RDA) for biotin, but the recommendation for adequate intake in adults is 30 micrograms (µg) per day, with more during pregnancy. Biotin is considered very safe. It is water-soluble, and excess amounts are excreted in the urine.[11]

Studies of biotin for MS have used a highly concentrated, pharmaceutical-grade version of the vitamin, referred to as MD1003. MD1003 is a mega-dose formulation containing 100 to 300 (sometimes 600) *milligrams* (mg) of biotin, which is about 10,000 times the commonly recommended daily dose of biotin from the diet, and about 300 times the usual supplement dose. Even such mega-doses seem to be well tolerated. High amounts of biotin appear to help promote myelin production, as well as improve the nerves' ability to send electrical signals. I take 100 mg three times a day as prescribed by my MS neurologist at Brigham and Women's Hospital in Boston.

In one small study of 23 people with progressive MS, 91 percent showed improvement within two to eight months of taking MD1003.[12] In a randomized, double-blind, placebo-controlled study of 154 people with primary and secondary progressive MS, those receiving MD1003 had significant improvement in their mobility as measured by a decrease on the Kurtzke Expanded Disability Status Scale (EDSS) compared with the placebo group. Improvement was still evident after two years. In fact, the number of people who improved on MD1003 actually increased as time went on, suggesting the need to stay on the treatment longer-term. In this study researchers estimated that participants who were given MD1003 had a 67 percent decreased risk of MS progression.[13] Two other randomized controlled studies found a slight improvement in progressive optic neuritis in people taking MD1003 compared with placebo.[14] And in an animal model of MS, MD1003 appeared to protect nerves in the spinal cord from demyelination.[15]

Most human studies of high-dose biotin for MS have shown positive results in improved function. As with many potential treatments, however, ongoing research is needed to understand the risks and benefits more fully. Not all evidence about high-dose biotin has been positive. One small study found that signs of inflammation increased, and that the average relapse rate almost tripled from the previous year during treatment with the mega-dose form of biotin.[16] Something else to be aware of is that biotin, sometimes even in low doses, can interfere with certain blood tests, leading to incorrect results. In particular, it can affect tests for thyroid function and heart function.[17] If you are taking biotin, always inform your health care provider if they are ordering blood work. If you take high doses of biotin, consider stopping it for a couple of days before a blood test.

Stem Cell Therapy

Stem cell therapy is being researched for its potential to slow down disease activity in people with aggressive forms of MS, as well as to repair nervous system damage. Currently, stem cell therapy is considered experimental and is not approved by the FDA for the treatment of MS in the United States. However, small clinical trials are starting to take place worldwide. While some initial findings are promising, the most recent study at the time of this writing showed no benefit.

Stem cells are present in a very early stage of physical development. Embryonic stem cells exist only at the earliest stages of development. They are *pluripotent*, which means they can become any cell type found in the body. Tissue-specific stem cells (also called *adult* or *somatic* stem cells), which arise during fetal development and remain in the body throughout life, are more specialized. Usually, this kind of stem cell creates the different cell types appropriate for the specific tissue or organ in which it is located. For example, hematopoietic (blood-forming) stem cells found in bone marrow can develop into red blood cells, white blood cells, and platelets, but not into liver cells or brain cells. And stem cells found in the liver and brain can't generate blood cells. Tissue-specific neural stem cells are found in the fetal and adult brain and spinal cord. These neural stem cells generate neurons, oligodendrocytes (myelin-producing cells), and astrocytes (nutritive and support cells for the brain). Another type of cell, the mesenchymal stem cell (MSC), is derived from bone marrow, blood, or fat cells, and can be manipulated in the laboratory to become cells that are found in very different organs and tissues.

Most stem cell research for MS has focused on achieving one of two outcomes. The first is finding ways to modulate the immune system to prevent attacks on myelin. Because immune cells that circulate in the blood are made in the bone marrow, a procedure known as hematopoietic stem cell transplant (HSCT) is being investigated as a means to restore a healthy immune response. This method involves transplanting stem cells isolated from bone marrow into patients with progressive types of MS, in the hope that the stem cells will reconstitute the patients' bone marrow and reboot a new, healthy immune system. Unfortunately, this procedure requires a temporary partial suppression, or even total destruction, of the recipient's immune system, which vastly raises the risk of life-threatening infections.

The second stem-based approach focuses on neuroregeneration—finding a way to turn stem cells into specialized cells that will stimulate repair of myelin damage that has already occurred. These cells would then be injected into the bloodstream or spinal fluid.

Interestingly, stem cell therapies in conjunction with the use of polyphenols like curcumin and resveratrol have shown a positive impact on inflammation in MS in laboratory models. Stem cell therapy is an exciting frontier for MS treatment. It holds some promise, especially to help with remyelination, but it is still in its early days. More clinical research needs to happen before we can understand how safe and effective it will be. There are patients who have died in stem cell clinics overseas, so beware. The National MS Society is a good resource for keeping up to date about ongoing studies of stem cell therapy.

Neuropeptides

Peptide therapy has been available in other parts of the world for many decades, but it's relatively new in the United States, where some peptide treatments have received FDA approval. As you may remember from high school science class, peptides are small chains of amino acids, which are the building blocks for proteins. Our body naturally produces an enormous array of peptides (around 300,000), and uses them to carry out almost every known (and not yet known!) complex biochemical process necessary for life. Peptide therapy is used to treat a wide range of symptoms, many of which are related to the negative consequences of aging. Many of the peptides used occur naturally, while others are manufactured in a laboratory setting. Injection is the most common form of delivery.

Peptides have been studied for their potential to help those with Alzheimer's disease, Parkinson's disease, and, increasingly, MS. Research suggests that some peptides may have protective and regenerative properties, acting in similar ways to NGF. These peptides appear able to shield neurons from inflammation and injury and to stimulate nerve regeneration. Some of the peptides that may prove promising for MS include:

Thymosin beta-4 (Tβ4), a synthetic peptide currently under investigation for a variety of applications, has been shown to increase brain cells known as oligodendrocyte progenitor cells, which support myelination. I take this product as an injection daily. It costs $400 per month, and I find it to be quite helpful. It is not covered by insurance.

Cerebrolysin is a parenterally (non-orally) administered drug that decreases deposition of amyloid plaque and increases levels of brain-derived neurotrophic factor (BDNF). Higher blood levels of BDNF are associated with improved cognitive functions.

BPC-157, which is a synthetic peptide originally synthesized from stomach acid, has been shown to promote remyelination of nerve cells following injury.

Glatiramer acetate (Copaxone), an FDA-approved drug, is a synthetic neuropeptide made from amino acids found in myelin that reduces relapse rates in relapsing-remitting multiple sclerosis. Glatiramer acetate has virtually no serious side effects, and has been shown to decrease MS attacks by 30 percent over two years. This is one of the first drugs used in the early stages of MS. I have taken it for 10 years as a daily injection, but was switched to Tecfidera for six months, and then switched to Ocrevus. It's hard to know what drugs are working; usually, as MS progresses, so must your treatment regimen.

A drawback to peptide therapy in general is that it is very expensive. In addition, many potentially helpful neuropeptides are currently available only to researchers. I want you to know about peptides, though, because they are an exciting frontier of medicine that may someday become more affordable (we can hope!) as well as more routinely prescribed for neurodegenerative and autoimmune conditions of all kinds.

CHAPTER 7

Regulating the Regulators

I n previous chapters, I've explained that research has established that multiple sclerosis involves inflammation in the brain and damage to the myelin sheath that protects nerve cells. And it's long been known that hormones play a key role in maintenance of brain and central nervous system (CNS) health. Putting this information together, it becomes clear that in order to effectively treat MS symptoms, it's important to understand the role of hormones in the body and how to achieve and maintain hormonal balance.

Hormones are substances produced and excreted by the human endocrine and nervous systems. Their job is to regulate body systems, from the digestive system to the reproductive, circulatory, respiratory, and nervous systems. You may not know the metabolic details of how hormones are produced and what they do. But chances are you are familiar with the names and basic actions of some common ones, including adrenaline, estrogen, testosterone, oxytocin, and melatonin. Melatonin, for example—also called the sleep hormone—reduces certain nerve activities in the brain and dopamine levels in the eyes, both of which help the body relax and prepare for rest.

Most hormones are produced in the endocrine system, a system of glands distributed throughout the body. Once produced, hormones enter the bloodstream and travel to their target sites, where they bind to specific receptors and exert some form of influence.

Hormone Production in the Brain, CNS, and Gut

The brain is part of the central nervous system, and it also acts as an endocrine organ. For example, the brain converts one type of hormone secreted by the thyroid gland into a more active form for the body's use (I describe this more fully later in this chapter). The brain has receptors for targeted endocrine hormones, and is part of an important feedback loop involving the pituitary gland (which regulates hormone production) and a variety of organs whose function depends upon those hormones. Consequently, the brain has the ability to direct and adjust bodily functions. It does so via production of neurotransmitters such as serotonin and dopamine. The brain and CNS also produce hormones known as neurosteroids. Synthesized from cholesterol, neurosteroids play a role in the myelination of neurons, as well as the growth, differentiation, and maintenance of neurons. (Because of cholesterol's importance in hormone production, I advise MS patients to think twice about using statins to lower their cholesterol levels. And because the human body manufactures cholesterol from fat, this is also why I advise including a variety of healthy fats in the diet—especially omega-3s, as discussed in chapter 5.)

Bacteria in the human microbiome also impact hormone production. In fact, gut bacteria produce almost 50 percent of the dopamine used by the body. The microbiome also impacts thyroid hormone conversion and the production of melatonin. This is why I adamantly recommend avoiding processed foods. Many of these may contain chemicals and preservatives that can disrupt hormone balance.

What Is the Neuroendocrine System?

Directed by the hypothalamus, the neuroendrocrine system regulates a variety of physiological processes, including metabolism, reproduction, blood pressure, and growth.[1]

Interestingly, new research suggests that "cross-talk" between the neuroendocrine and immune systems could be responsible for regulating the body's response to injury and inflammation, which could help us better understand how certain diseases of the CNS develop.[2]

How Hormones Do Their Work

Hormones serve two functions: messaging and the regulation of body systems. In some cases a pair of hormones work in a kind of feedback loop. When this happens, Hormone X acts as a messenger to stimulate or depress an endocrine gland in response to the body's needs. That gland then releases either more or less of a second hormone, Hormone Y.

When thyroid hormone levels in the body reach normal levels, the brain receives another message through the feedback loop. The brain calls upon the pituitary gland to slow its release of thyroid-stimulating hormone (TSH). The reduction of TSH in the bloodstream signals the thyroid gland to slow the release of thyroid hormone.

When working properly, feedback loops help ensure that cells have the proper amount of necessary hormones at all times, keeping the body in balance. But sometimes those loops can lose their balance, causing too little or too much of a hormone to be released, which can result in damage to cells and tissues. Even worse, a domino effect can occur, triggering imbalances in other hormones. which can lead to other interrelated health problems.

The Impact of Aging on Hormones

As we age, hormone production naturally declines, causing physical and psychological changes in both men and women. The pace at which hormones decline, and thus the rate at which we age, are determined by our genetic makeup, lifestyle, diet choices, exercise levels, weight/BMI, stress level, relationship status, community involvement, and other factors. For example, common life situations such as smoking or gaining excessive weight can cause testosterone production to decline faster.[3] The stress related to job loss or divorce can increase cortisol levels and cause weight gain and damage to neurons. In women, the precipitous drop in estrogen due to age combined with the fact that females tend to have longer life expectancy than males means that women generally experience more cognitive changes with age and have higher rates of Alzheimer's disease than men.

Many other factors influence the complex aging process, and aging is the result of the accumulation of factors, not a single hormonal change.[4]

The Role of Hormones in MS and Other Neurodegenerative Diseases

Over the short and the long term, hormones can have both positive and negative effects on the health of the brain and the central nervous system. One example is the effect of hormones on neurons in multiple sclerosis.

Although their actions are not well understood, neurosteroid hormones can help to mitigate the severity and the progression of MS. They do so by influencing oligodendrocytes to provide neuroprotection and remyelination that reduces and repairs damage to the myelin sheath.

To date, many of the studies examining the connections between hormones and neurodegenerative disease have focused on Alzheimer's— which is why I reference studies on Alzheimer's quite often in this chapter. Although research into hormones and MS is relatively young, the implications are similar.

Thyroid Hormones

The thyroid produces two hormones, T3 and T4, that regulate the body's metabolic rate and other elements of health, including breathing, heart rate, central and peripheral nervous systems, body weight, muscle strength, menstrual cycles, body temperature, and cholesterol levels. Thyroid hormones also support proper central nervous system function and interact with many facets of the nervous system to help prevent dementia. Maturation of oligodendrocytes and myelination is influenced by thyroid hormone (TH) signaling. Thyroid hormone interacts with acetylcholine, which, as mentioned previously, improves memory and prevents cognitive decline. Low thyroid hormone status can cause insufficient production of acetylcholine. Research has shown that patients with Alzheimer's disease have diminishing levels of acetylcholine relative to the progression of the disease.[5]

Triiodothyronine (also called T3) and thyroxine (also called T4) are two hormones that are critical for normal metabolic functioning. Most (about 80 percent) of T3, known as the active thyroid hormone, results from *deiodination*—the process by which organs such as the liver and kidneys remove one of the four iodine molecules that are part of T4. Some inactive thyroid

Hormones and Cognition

Changes in hormone levels can cause a range of cognitive symptoms, including:

- Losing your train of thought, having trouble prioritizing tasks, and other disturbances in linear thinking
- Having to rely on "filler" phrases, such as "you know what I mean," in conversation, and other changes in speech
- Taking longer to retrieve memories; doing so with less accuracy; trouble recalling recent events; and other short- and long-term memory impacts

hormone results from this process as well; that hormone is called reverse T3, or rT3. The thyroid gland produces the other 20 percent of T3 (by combining dietary iodine with the amino acid tyrosine) as well as all of T4.

T3, the active thyroid hormone, promotes nerve growth factor (NGF). (As described in chapter 6, NGF supports nerve growth, proliferation, function, and nerve myelination.) T3 also enhances remyelination by supporting oligodendrocyte precursor cells (OPCs). Without adequate thyroid hormone, there is a deficiency of mature, active OPCs and limited ability for myelin repair.[6]

The brain is extremely dependent on thyroid hormone. Low thyroid levels are believed to cause shrinking of the hippocampus, the part of the brain that shifts short-term memories to long-term, enables spatial memory related to navigation, and supports memory and learning. The hippocampus is particularly significant because it is the part of the brain that shows the earliest signs of damage in Alzheimer's disease (AD) patients. When present in adequate amounts, thyroid hormones may help ward off dementia by hindering a protein that promotes amyloid production and indirectly prevents plaque deposits. On the other hand, deficient thyroid levels may open the floodgates for more amyloid production and consequent damage to the brain.[7]

Adults who develop hypothyroidism can suffer from poor memory, confusion, and difficulty learning new tasks. Fortunately, these symptoms are reversible in adult hypothyroidism, simply by restoring thyroid hormone levels and body temperature.

Thyroid hormone may indirectly contribute to dementia through its influence on the cardiovascular system. Hypothyroidism is a significant risk factor for developing cardiovascular disease. In this condition, blood flow to the brain may become impaired due to a compromised vascular system. Diminished blood flow and the resulting poor delivery of oxygen and nutrients to the brain can contribute to damage in the brain and an increased risk of developing AD.[8]

Thyroid hormone is so crucial to the brain that if there is inadequate thyroid hormone available to a fetus developing in the womb, its brain and neurons will not mature properly, causing irreversible mental deficiencies in the form of cretinisim.

A very large clinical trial conducted by Boston University in collaboration with the National Heart, Lung, and Blood Institute known as the Framingham Study collected health data on almost 2,000 people over the course of nearly 13 years to better learn about risk factors for various diseases. It found that for women with non-normal TSH levels (which is an indicator of either elevated or deficient thyroid hormone), there was more than *double* the risk of developing AD as for women with healthy normal levels.[9]

Therapeutic Use for MS

MS patients are shown to have higher rates of thyroid disorders as compared with healthy peers. One study showed that patients with MS had a significantly higher risk of also having *autoimmune* thyroid disease, specifically Graves' disease (hyperthyroidism) and Hashimoto's disease (hypothyroidism).[10] I mention this here because individuals with one autoimmune condition are more susceptible to developing others—which could explain the correlation between MS and these types of thyroid disease.

Animal research has shown that daily injections of T3, the active form of thyroid hormone, contributes to remyelination. These studies also show that thyroid hormone supplementation can improve neurological symptoms in animals and improve proliferation and activation of OPC.[11] At Oregon Health and

Science University, thyroid hormone is being studied as a potential MS therapy due to its critical role in protecting myelin and promoting remyelination.

T3 supplementation is not standard of care for MS, but I have found it one of the top three significant therapies in treating my own fatigue and brain fog. When demyelination occurs during an MS attack, the body does produce more rT3, which blocks the active T3 hormone from working. Reverse T3 slows the activity of metabolism in the body and the CNS. It is a normal function to slow metabolic processes during times of fasting, to conserve energy, and also during times of grief. However when the rT3 stays high for the long term, this otherwise healthy slowing process can persist to the point that it leads to chronic disease. It is analogous in this way to inflammation—an appropriate amount of inflammation helps tissues heal, but excess can be damaging. In the case of rT3, overly high levels can contribute to significant, debilitating fatigue. Adding T3 to the body can help take the edge off the fatigue that MS patients experience, especially after an attack, and help the mind become clearer. Interestingly, thyroid hormones stimulate myelination.

Every couple of years, I take 5 mcg of T3 twice a day for a three-month period. This dosage has a beneficial effect for me. I also take a product that I formulated myself called Thyroid Px. This supplement combines iodine, selenium, and thyroid-activating herbs. Over time, my MRI scans have shown some lesions to decrease in size and some to disappear. Although I cannot know for sure, because some types of MS lesions do heal on their own over time, I attribute the size reduction and disappearance of some of my lesions in part to the body's natural ability to heal itself and in part to the restorative treatments I take.

Estrogen

Estrogens are a family of hormones that includes estrone, estradiol (the most abundant), and estriol (the mildest form of estrogen, produced during pregnancy). Known as the primary sex hormones for women, estrogens are related to reproduction and bone density, but also have significant effects on the brain and CNS. Neurons have estrogen receptors, which can enhance nerve growth factor to help protect cells from neurodegeneration.[12]

Testing and Tracking Hormones

Because hormones are integral to brain health, one effective strategy in your MS treatment tool kit is to test and track their levels. Any integrative medicine practitioner (one who uses a holistic approach to healing) can do this for you.

Regarding thyroid testing, I am one of the growing body of practitioners who believe the standard tests, including the test for the level of TSH in a blood sample, can be deceptive. That is, even though such test results register as normal, patients can still exhibit symptoms indicating otherwise.

Be sure to inform your doctor if you experience more than one symptom of hypothyroidism, such as chronic fatigue, unexplained weight gain, depression, constipation, or consistently low body temperature, because you may have subclinical hypothyroidism. In such cases, treatment with thyroid hormone can improve symptoms and protect your brain's health.

Of course, it's important to find an experienced naturopathic doctor or integrative medicine specialist who can help you determine whether hormone therapy is right for you.

Estrogen promotes nerve growth, modulates the immune system to reduce autoimmune reactions, and promotes the repair of brain cells when they are damaged. Estrogen can also enhance blood flow, and thus oxygen and nutrient delivery to the brain.[13] Estrogen is the hormonal factor that enhances women's verbal memory, fluency, and language.

Estrogen seems to influence the severity of MS symptoms. The third trimester of pregnancy, when estriol levels in women are highest, is associated with a 70 percent reduction in MS relapse rates. MS relapses tend to increase after pregnancy, when estrogen levels drop, and disease progression resumes as well. While the reason for these changes is uncertain, estrogen is believed to influence immune activity—perhaps because symptoms of other autoimmune diseases, such as rheumatoid arthritis and psoriasis, also decline during pregnancy.[14]

In addition, estrogen protects nerves; helps clear beta-amyloid; and influences the brain's production of serotonin, acetylcholine, noradrenaline, and other neurotransmitters. The release of such neurotransmitters can influence mood and emotions. Extensive research has been conducted to better understand the complex interplay of hormones such as estrogen and neurotransmitters, but there is still much to learn.[15]

Therapeutic Use for MS

Estrogen may be one of the most studied hormones, but don't be fooled. The story of estrogen and the role of estrogen hormone therapy is neither simple nor straightforward.

Estrogen is known to have a protective effect on nerve growth, myelination, the hippocampus, and general brain health. With aging in both men and women, estrogen levels drop and its protective action declines, although hormone treatment can stabilize levels and increase protection.[16]

Women experience higher rates of MS and other autoimmune diseases than men, particularly earlier in life. The reasons why are unclear, but young men have higher levels of testosterone than older men do, and testosterone may have a protective effect. Yet surprisingly, men who do have MS tend to have a significantly more severe disease course than women.

Women also have a higher risk for developing Alzheimer's disease than men. This is believed to be linked to the abrupt decline of estrogen that occurs with menopause, and thus the loss of its neuroprotective, immunomodulating, and anti-inflammatory effects.[17] Estrogen also has an antioxidant action. Because of this, there's a temptation to assume that estrogen treatment would automatically help alleviate neurodegenerative diseases such as MS and AD. While this is true in some cases, research has demonstrated that the specific form of estrogen and the timing for starting treatment are critical factors for treating MS and AD.

Estriol is thought to be the most beneficial of the estrogens for MS. Animal studies show that estriol repairs brain cells by maintaining healthy neuron synapses and causing immune changes that reduce the impact of autoimmune diseases.[18] In a two-year clinical study, 164 women with relapsing-remitting

MS participated in a trial using a combination therapy of oral estriol or placebo in addition to a standard MS drug. The group of women taking the estriol combination showed a significant reduction in relapse rate compared with the women who did not take the hormone. But there were no significant differences in other measurements, such as number and size of brain lesions or degree of disability. The researchers concluded that the results were promising, but that larger studies would be required to determine whether estriol treatment is beneficial.[19] Oral contraceptives, which are composed of synthetic estrogens and without estriol, have not been shown to be effective in preventing MS, reducing relapses, or improving symptoms.[20]

Whether estrogen therapy provides brain protection is, surprisingly, still debatable and requires more research. In a study published in 2017 that reviewed 22 clinical trials focused on tracking postmenopausal women taking long-term hormone replacement therapy (HRT), the overall conclusion was that long-term hormone therapy did not provide the same protective effects that natural estrogen offers. In fact, long-term use of estrogen-only and combined-estrogen-and-progesterone treatment was shown to increase a woman's risk of stroke, heart attack, and gallbladder disease. Women taking combined hormone therapy also showed an increased risk of dementia. In this review, the only benefits shown for hormone therapy were preventing fractures and alleviating menopause symptoms.[21]

A clinical trial from Finland published in 2017 also showed mixed results regarding the brain-protecting effects of HRT. This very large study reviewed over a decade's worth of health data from the medical files of more than 200,000 women. The reviewers found that women who took estrogen, progesterone, or a combination of the two for fewer than 10 years had an increased risk of AD. But taking estrogen-only for over 10 years lowered their risk of developing AD, while progesterone alone or combined with estrogen showed no changes in AD risk. It was also found that for women over 75 years of age, HRT offered no brain-protective benefits. The overall conclusion from these researchers was that HRT use does not significantly influence future AD risk.[22]

The results of these studies may seem confusing or contradictory. This may be due to differences in timing of treatments and type of hormones used. There is a theory about a "critical window" for starting HRT to treat AD—that in order to provide protective benefits, HRT must be started very shortly after estrogen levels plummet during menopause and long before there are changes in cognitive function. If HRT is started after changes in the brain have started to develop, the therapy may actually have a detrimental effect.[23] In the previously cited studies, the women most likely took synthetic estrogen and progesterone of the types most commonly prescribed, such as Premarin and progestin. One small clinical study showed that topical (transdermal) estrogen combined with progesterone helped decrease amyloid deposits in the brain when treatment was initiated shortly after onset of menopause. Two other groups in the study took either oral hormone replacement or placebo; neither of those groups showed any effect on amyloid deposits. Although this study was small, it suggests the possibility that transdermal HRT may be a more promising treatment than oral HRT, and it confirmed the notion that timing for initiating treatment is a critical factor for success.[24] More research is needed to confirm if it actually is effective in neuroprotection and to explore the best types of hormone delivery systems and determine the most appropriate timing.

As for men who have MS, I would not recommend estriol unless they want to develop female characteristics such as enlarged breasts. For women, I would consider trying a low dose of estriol as a therapeutic trial that is overseen by their prescribing doctor.

Progesterone

New research indicates that progesterone is produced not only in the ovaries, but also by neurons, and thus it is a neurosteroid. Progesterone made by neurons promotes dendritic growth and possibly myelin repair. Regardless of where it is made, therefore, progesterone and its metabolite, allopregnanolone, show promise as potential treatments for neurodegenerative disorders, but more research is required.[25]

Progesterone, like estrogen, is most notable for its role in reproduction and pregnancy. Recent research has revealed that progesterone has a significant neuroendocrine role. This may lead to important contributions in the prevention of neurodegenerative diseases. Studies show that when progesterone is converted to active metabolites, specifically allopregnanolone, it can act on neurons to promote myelin repair.

Therapeutic Use for MS

Progesterone and allopregnanolone have been shown in animal studies to be anti-inflammatory and protective of myelin.[26] No human clinical studies have been conducted at the time of this writing. Treating with progestins, the synthetic version of progesterone, as of yet has not been shown clinically beneficial in protecting myelin, but natural, bioidentical progesterone may offer better results, and deserves further research.[27]

Testosterone

Testosterone, the primary male sex hormone, is responsible for sex drive, bone and muscle building, fat distribution, and red blood cell production. It is present in women, but in smaller quantities than in men. In the body testosterone is metabolized to dihydrotestosterone (DHT) and estradiol, which complicates understanding its effects.

Testosterone and DHT have several important functions related to cognition. The brain has receptors for testosterone in specific areas such as the hippocampus. Testosterone also stimulates nerve differentiation and enhances nerve communication.[28]

Testosterone, like estrogen, influences specific cognitive skills. For example, men—and women with above-normal testosterone levels—have better spatial cognition, navigation skills, and spatial memory (which are important for tasks such as handling tools or dancing) than people whose bodies are more heavily influenced by estrogen.

When testosterone levels are deficient, arteries in the brain weaken, predisposing a person to stroke or clots. In compromised vessels, blood flow is diminished and oxygen and nutrient delivery is insufficient, contributing to poor memory and cognition.

Therapeutic Use for MS

The relationship between testosterone levels and neurodegenerative diseases such as MS and AD is unclear and underexplored. Several studies support the theory that testosterone levels are lower than normal in men with MS, and one study showed that women with MS have significantly lower levels of testosterone than healthy women.[29] Some, but not all, studies show a pattern of lower testosterone levels in men with AD as compared with men without AD. It is theorized that similar to estrogen, testosterone may play a role in preventing amyloid-beta from accumulating, and when hormone levels decline, that protection is lost.[30]

Research on testosterone treatment for neurological diseases such as MS is limited, and the results are conflicting. There is some in vitro evidence that testosterone reduces inflammation, but it is less clear whether testosterone is neuroprotective. One study showed that giving the testosterone metabolite DHT to animals helped reduce neuroinflammation and had a protective antioxidant effect.[31]

Testosterone shows some neuroprotective effects in how it interacts with the hippocampus to benefit memory.[32] In a clinical study, administration of testosterone in men with Alzheimer's disease helped improve spatial memory and overall life quality, but did not affect other aspects of AD.[33]

Much more research is needed to better understand the role of testosterone on the brain and nerves and how it can be applied therapeutically. Personally based on the limited research, I would only recommend testosterone supplementation if someone is low in it.

Pregnenolone

Known as the mother hormone, pregnenolone is created from cholesterol and is the building block for other hormones such as testosterone, progesterone, and estrogen.[34] It is produced in the adrenal glands, ovaries, testes, and even the central nervous system. Because it serves as a precursor to other hormones, pregnenolone is the most abundant of all hormones in the brain. Scientists have discovered that in certain ways, pregnenolone acts similarly to a neurotransmitter, and that it can improve memory, support concentration, enhance clear thinking, and prevent memory loss.

Therapeutic Use for MS

Pregnenolone levels vary in MS depending on the type and stage of disease. Men with relapsing-remitting MS have been shown to have elevated levels of pregnenolone.[35]

Pregnenolone levels generally decline with age in both men and women. This decline seems to play a role in dementia. Because it is the mother hormone from which many other brain-influencing hormones are cre-ated, pregnenolone deficit can indirectly but significantly affect the brain. Pregnenolone also activates switches in the brain that enhance the brain's communication network and provide neuroprotection.[36]

The relationship between pregnenolone and dementia is further con-firmed by the finding that AD patients have lower levels of pregnenolone and its metabolite allopregnanolone in the brain than healthy peers.[37] The relationship is also supported by animal studies, which have shown that administering pregnenolone has an immediate memory-boosting effect.[38] Research is required to determine whether pregnenolone supplementation is beneficial for preventing or treating dementia.

I take a product that I formulated called Adrenal Px DHEA, which com-bines pregnenolone and dehydroepiandrosterone (DHEA)—a hormone produced in the adrenal gland that helps produce other hormones, including testosterone and estrogen. Because DHEA levels peak in early adulthood, supplementing with it theoretically can address some common complaints associated with aging. It can also address symptoms of adrenal insufficiency and fatigue. My formulation does help with my energy, but doesn't seem to affect any other symptoms.

Cortisol

Cortisol, also known as the stress hormone, is secreted by the adrenal glands. Levels naturally rise in the morning, which rouses us out of sleep; levels then decrease throughout the day until we go to sleep. When balanced, cortisol works with various bodily systems to reduce inflammation, regulate blood pressure, increase blood sugar levels, and help maintain a regular sleep cycle. It is the hormone secreted in response to stressful events, both emotional and physical. It's one of the fight-or-flight hormones that are secreted to give the body an extreme burst of energy in reaction to a life-or-death situation. Cor-tisol secretion can also be triggered by emotional situations, such as feeling lonely or socially embarrassed.[39]

Cortisol essentially controls motivation, fear, and even mood. As with other hormones, it works on a feedback loop; when the brain gets the mes-sage that blood cortisol levels are too low for normal function, the brain signals the adrenal system to secrete more. And as with other hormones, balance is critical when it comes to cortisol. Ongoing stress can elevate cortisol levels, causing health problems such as heart disease, poor memory and concentration, insomnia, and weight gain. Chronic excess cortisol also causes the hippocampus to shrink, changes the way that neurons mature, and can irreversibly make neurons less efficient and useful. The consequence is inhibited communication between different parts of the brain.[40] Not surprisingly, studies show that chronically elevated cortisol levels are associated with accelerated aging and diminished cognitive function in older adults.

Contrary to the pattern of other hormones, cortisol levels rise naturally as we get older. One of the contributing factors may be that older people have a more significant cortisol response or sensitivity to stress than younger adults. This reaction is particularly higher for older women.

One explanation for this increased cortisol sensitivity is that older adults have been shown to have smaller hippocampus volume. It's still not clear if this brain-shrinking phenomenon is caused by excess cortisol, or if it is the cause of increased cortisol secretion. Studies show that for older adults, a lower threshold of stress will trigger a decline in memory performance. Younger people, however, can tolerate much higher levels of stress without memory impairment due to their larger hippocampus volume. Elevated cortisol levels in older adults eventually causes damage to the brain and other body systems, increasing the likelihood of development of memory problems commonly seen in the elderly.

Research shows that older patients with dementia have an imbalance of the hypothalamic-pituitary-adrenal (HPA) axis, leading to excess cortisol secretion.[41]

Aging and stress are not the only cause for high cortisol levels. A disease of the adrenals called Cushing's disease causes chronic excess cortisol secretion. It has been found that patients with Cushing's disease often suffer from brain atrophy and reduced cognitive skills due to cortisol overexposure.[42]

Further proof that cortisol impacts cognitive function has been revealed by looking at the side effects of cortisone. Cortisone, the pharmaceutical version of cortisol, is used as an anti-inflammatory treatment for joint conditions and other problems. Soon after cortisone was developed and tested, researchers became aware that it had effects similar to the excessive volumes compared with controls.[43]

Therapeutic Use for MS

Solu-Medrol (methylprednisolone) is an intravenous (IV) form of prednisone (a type of corticosteroid). In MS patients, it's commonly used to treat acute, symptomatic flares; in this case, a health care provider administers 1,000 mg intravenously each day for three to five days. I have only taken prednisone after a serious attack, and it did alleviate some of my symptoms, including tachycardia (fast heart rate) and my loss of ability to walk. For some cortisone users, side effects include mental disturbances such as anxiety, poor memory and concentration, and other brain-related problems.[44] Patients taking long-term oral corticosteroids/cortisone have been shown to have smaller hippocampal volume, but this has not been shown to positively affect long-term disability and, surprisingly, it has no impact on MS progression. I find like many other MS patients taking this treatment that IV prednisone keeps me awake at night. And a more serious consequence of long-term steroid use is that it can cause osteoporosis. But when I do need to take prednisone, I ask to take it as early in the morning as possible. This provides the best chance that it will not adversely affect my sleep. I also take 6 mg of melatonin mixed in with valerian and hops during the evening of these IV drips. I take this in the form of commercial capsules called Sleep (that's the product name) just before bedtime.

Although many conventional physicians do raise an eyebrow at my treatments, including low doses of 5 mg of hydrocortisone at noon to help with energy, such doses do not impact blood tests, and do not suppress the HPA axis. MS patients do tend to have lower levels of cortisol, which might predispose them to attacks. I do this treatment for no more than three months a year. It is important to recognize that this is very different from taking Solu-Medrol.

Melatonin

Melatonin is produced primarily by the pineal gland in the brain, although the gastrointestinal tract and immune cells also secrete melatonin. Melatonin maintains our circadian rhythm, also known as the sleep-wake cycle. Melatonin levels peak at night to induce sleep; its levels are lowest in daylight. Melatonin levels decline naturally with age, which may help explain why older adults have more sleep problems than younger adults.

People with multiple sclerosis also have sleep problems and resulting fatigue. This is attributed to lower-than-normal melatonin levels. It's not clear if low melatonin level is a risk factor for developing MS. One large study of night-shift workers showed that working at night, which alters natural melatonin secretion, increases the risk of developing MS.[45]

Some research suggests that melatonin production is decreased in patients with MS, which may be due to pineal gland dysfunction.

For some people with MS, like me, the flaring up of symptoms and frequency of relapse are known to have seasonal variability, whereby symptoms are more likely to flare up in the spring and summer than the fall and winter. Melatonin levels are lower in spring and summer in northern climates (where the incidence of MS is greater), and some studies suggest that the decreased disease activity of MS observed in autumn and winter might have something to do with the naturally higher levels of melatonin people experience at those times.

Melatonin is also a powerful antioxidant as well as being neuroprotective. It has been shown to reduce the formation of beta-amyloid plaques and may support production of the neurotransmitter acetylcholine, thus making it an important hormone for the regulation of memory and cognition. Melatonin has been shown to decrease symptom severity and behavioral deficits in animal models of MS. Studies have also shown that people with Alzheimer's disease and Parkinson's disease have abnormalities in their melatonin production.

Therapeutic Use in MS

Most research on the impact of melatonin treatment for MS has been in vitro or animal research. In MS animal models, high-dose melatonin is shown to improve disease symptoms.[46] One clinical trial in humans examined the use of melatonin for patients with MS. Melatonin was shown to have a significant antioxidative effect, but it did not significantly improve symptoms of fatigue.[47] Melatonin has a complicated relationship with autoimmune diseases but seems to be beneficial for MS. For example, MS patients generally experience an improvement in symptoms in fall and winter, when days are shorter and melatonin levels in the body tend to be higher.

In vitro studies show that melatonin can dampen the autoimmune response and have a protective effect.[48] Melatonin is also known to be a potent antioxidant, and excessive oxidative stress may be a factor in the progression of MS.[49]

More research is necessary to determine possible benefits of melatonin supplementation.

———

As all of the above makes clear, a balanced endocrine system is essential for a healthy brain. In addition to hormone treatments, you can use complementary strategies—following a healthy diet, maintaining an appropriate weight and BMI ratio, getting proper sleep, managing stress, and indulging in mindfulness practices—to achieve that balance. Please refer to the appropriate sections of this book for more information about, and my personal experiences with, using these strategies.

CHAPTER 8

The Great Communicators

The field of neurodegenerative disease is complicated, and much remains to be learned through research. As I've explained in previous chapters, there are two ways to address neurodegenerative diseases: neuroprotection and neurorestoration.[1] The more effective, of course, is through neuroprotection—that is, preventing damage to the nervous system and maintaining its health. This requires a better understanding of the nervous system in order to anticipate imbalances before symptoms develop and the imbalances develop into full-blown disease. In addition, research may identify natural compounds and medicines that protect the nervous system from oxidation and neuroinflammation and prevent disease progression.

Neurorestoration calls for repairing neurons after neurodegeneration becomes obvious through symptoms. For many diseases, neurorestorative treatments have a much lower rate of success. But they do show some early promise for MS.

You'll recall from chapter 1 that the myelin sheath wraps around and protects the axons, which are responsible for sending electrical signals from the brain. When myelin and axons experience damage, transmission dysfunctions occur within the CNS, causing many of the physical and cognitive symptoms I've covered elsewhere. This might explain why therapies leveraging specific neurotransmitters have shown some encouraging neuroprotective and neurorestorative effects.

In this chapter I'll delve into the research on some specific neurotransmitters, their role in maintaining healthy functioning of the body and mind, and their implications in MS. In order to set the stage, I first need to cover how nerve impulses are generated and transmitted in the body, and where neurotransmitters fit in.

The Role of Neurotransmitters

Neurotransmitters are chemical messengers that are critical to the ability of neurons to communicate with one another. Without delving too deeply into the science of it, which can be somewhat complicated, their mode of action goes something like this:

Neurons (and some other types of cells) synthesize neurotransmitters, which are then stored in small sacs (called *vesicles*) that essentially "hang out" near the ends of axons. In response to specific sensory stimuli, an electrical signal (called an *action potential*) travels down the length of a nerve to its axon, where it triggers the release of those neurotransmitters at the *presynaptic terminal*. (Recall that the synapse is the gap between the axon of one nerve and the dendrite of another.) Much as a boat can ferry passengers across a canal, neurotransmitters carry the action potential across the synapse, where they

Key Neurotransmitters

Acetylcholine. Can be excitatory or inhibitory. Stimulates muscle contraction along with many other functions.

GABA. Inhibitory to the central nervous system and has a calming action.

Dopamine. Can be excitatory or inhibitory. Especially prominent for reward-motivated behavior.

Serotonin (5-hydroxytryptamine). Inhibitory and regulates mood.

Glutamate. Excitatory, can be neurotoxic in excess.

Histamine. Can be excitatory or inhibitory.

Epinephrine and *norepinephrine.* Excitatory; related to the fight-or-flight reaction.

"dock" on the *postsynaptic terminal* with help from receptor cells ready to bind to them. Once docked, the neurotransmitters activate these receptors, which sparks another action potential. Stated slightly more simply, neurotransmitters take an electrical signal, convert it into a chemical one in order to cross the synapse, and then switch the signal back to an electrical one. Ultimately, these signals may travel to other body parts and exert a specific response.

Types of Neurotransmitters

Neurotransmitters essentially fall into one of two categories—*excitatory* and *inhibitory*. Excitatory neurotransmitters can trigger action potential. They include glutamate, epinephrine, and norepinephrine. Inhibitory neurotransmitters can inhibit action potential. They include γ-aminobutyric acid (GABA), glycine, and serotonin. Neurotransmitters are complex, however, and don't always fit into just one category. Some have both inhibitory and excitatory effects, depending on the conditions or existing receptors. To further complicate the story, some neurotransmitters may also have hormonal actions.

Neurotransmitter imbalances occur because of low production or because they are metabolized or broken down too quickly by enzymes. In a healthy state, key neurotransmitters exist in a specific ratio to balance one another. Imbalances can cause a wide variety of health problems such as fatigue, pain, insomnia, depression, and neurodegeneration.

Serotonin

If ever there was a "popular" neurotransmitter, it would be serotonin. It's one of the best-known neurotransmitters, although it's also considered a hormone under some conditions. It's often called the happy hormone, due to its association with a pleasant mood.

Serotonin, known also by its scientific name 5-hydroxytryptamine (5-HT), resides primarily in the gastrointestinal system, but is also found to a lesser degree in the nervous system and in blood platelets. When in balance, serotonin helps regulate appetite, emotions, sexual function, and cognition. It also has an indirect impact on the nervous system and motor functions.

Serotonin is the precursor for melatonin, which means it indirectly helps regulate a consistent sleep-wake schedule.

Researchers believe that depression is caused by a deficiency or imbalance of serotonin. As mentioned previously, depression is a common symptom in neurodegenerative disorders such as multiple sclerosis, Parkinson's disease, and Alzheimer's disease (AD). This may be so in part because these diseases can *cause* serotonin imbalances. The prescription drugs used to treat depression mainly target biochemical pathways to increase serotonin levels.[2]

Like other neurotransmitters, serotonin aids communication between neurons. It regulates bowel function and suppresses appetite. Because it resides in platelets, it can help promote clot formation, which helps wounds to heal. Despite serotonin's nickname of the happy hormone, side effects of increasing serotonin through medication include lower libido and poor sexual performance. The appeal of recreational drugs such as ecstasy and LSD is due in part to their ability to elevate serotonin, causing a pleasurable sensation.

Serotonin is produced in nerve cells from the essential amino acid tryptophan. Tryptophan is found in foods high in protein, including meat, salmon, soy, eggs, nuts, and cheese. Light therapy, exercise, and increasing tryptophan levels through diet can enhance serotonin levels.

As with many other hormones, serotonin levels decline progressively with age. A study from Johns Hopkins showed that older people with mild cognitive decline had lower levels of serotonin compared with their peers with normal brain function. Lower serotonin levels also coincide with lower scores on memory tests.[3]

Serotonin and the Gastrointestinal Tract

Serotonin is primarily found in the gastrointestinal tract (GI). For that reason, it is a major factor in the gut-brain axis. The health of the GI sets the tone for mood and anxiety. When the microbial environment in the GI is off balance, it can lead to serotonin imbalance and consequent mood disorders. Conversely, changes in the environment, such as conditions of extreme stress, can negatively influence the microbial health of the GI. Preliminary research shows that giving probiotics to people with depression and anxiety can improve their symptoms and reduce their anxiety, but this seems to be true only while ingestion of probiotics continues.[4] As mentioned in chapter 3, taking probiotic supplements impacts gut flora only temporarily; ingesting probiotics does not create a new healthy microbiome that perpetuates itself on its own.

The microbiome also influences neurodegenerative diseases. Alzheimer's disease research shows that adjusting the bacterial composition (using short-chain fatty acids or probiotics) in the GI can improve memory and slow amyloid plaque progression.[5]

Also related to the gastrointestinal tract is constipation—a common symptom in MS. Medications that increase serotonin may be beneficial for GI motility and preventing sluggish bowels. The reason these medications are beneficial is because there are serotonin receptors in the gut that can trigger acetylcholine release. This stimulates movement in the colon. For more information on medications to treat constipation, see the "Bladder and Bowel Health" section in chapter 9.

Serotonin and MS

Serotonin is one of the most studied neurotransmitters in the field of multiple sclerosis research. The amino acid tryptophan tends to be too low in patients with MS, which may contribute to lower serotonin production. Brain serotonin levels have been shown to be low in patients with MS. The production and metabolism of both serotonin and melatonin are reduced. The imbalance of serotonin may contribute to mental symptoms such as fatigue and depression, both of which are common and frustrating symptoms for MS patients. The lower the serotonin levels drop, the worse the symptoms of fatigue become.

Selective serotonin reuptake inhibitor medications (SSRIs) have the effect of increasing serotonin availability. Although it has not yet been proven, SSRIs show potential to reduce the formation of new lesions in MS. Studies also show that taking SSRIs can minimize stress-related relapses in MS. One research study tracked the health outcomes for MS patients who took SSRIs as compared with those who did not. The goal was to determine whether antidepressant medications significantly altered the progression of disease over time. This study did not find a significant protective effect for the SSRI fluoxetine (Prozac) in terms of MS disability and disease progression.[6] In contrast, other studies—both animal and human—found that fluoxetine could prevent neuronal damage in MS and positively influence the immune system in order to help prevent inflammatory lesions and slow disease progression.[7] The jury is still out; longer and larger studies are needed to determine whether fluoxetine can effectively slow progression of MS.

Lab tests to determine neurotransmitter levels can be helpful in determining the needs of a patient. MS patients who test low in serotonin and are experiencing depression might find relief by taking the serotonin precursor 5-HTP at doses of 200 mg per day.

Rhodiola Effect on Serotonin

Rhodiola rosea is another adaptogenic herb that is very powerful in supporting a healthy stress response, as well as all the benefits that go along with that, such as improved sleep and cognitive functions like memory and attention. Rhodiola roots contain a group of bioactive constituents known collectively as *salidrosides*. Rhodiola, and especially its salidrosides, may protect neurons from beta-amyloid plaque, regulate production of acetylcholine, and support neuronal repair. Rhodiola is also a potent antioxidant and may protect nerve cells through that mechanism as well. In animal studies it increased 5-HTP (serotonic precursor) in the hippocampus.

I source rhodiola harvested in Canada and Alaska rather than the one wildcrafted in Asia, where it is becoming endangered. I drink it as a tea, or ingest it as a capsule with a product I designed called Adrenal Px Balance. The rhodiola root is traditionally called roseroot, because it has a rose-fragranced flavor that's delicious. Most of these herbs can be helpful in maintaining energy, and can be more nourishing than coffee.

Acetylcholine

People who have neurological disorders in general exhibit low levels of the neurotransmitter acetylcholine (ACh). You'll notice that many of my recommendations below impact acetylcholine regulation, which is by design. Acetylcholine is one of the peripheral nervous system's primary neurotransmitters and is crucial to modulating overall brain function. Further, research has shown that when acetylcholine synthesis malfunctions, a variety of neurological pathologies, including neuroinflammation, can result.

As mentioned earlier in the book, one way to try to increase acetylcholine is by taking holy basil, which can increase levels of choline acetyltransferase

(ChAT), which helps the body *make* acetylcholine. Another approach is to try to *lower* levels of a substance whose job it is to *break down* acetylcholine. That substance is called acetylcholinesterase (AChE).

In MS it is possible that a high level of AChE is the primary cause of low acetylcholine levels. This kind of imbalance also promotes the production of inflammatory immune cells. An interesting study that used a computer model to simulate the biochemistry of human nerve cells determined that withanolide A (found in ashwagandha, which, as discussed earlier in the book, shows neuroprotective activity) might be able to inhibit production of AChE, thus boosting levels of acetylcholine for patients with MS, Alzheimer's disease, and potentially other neurological disorders.

Acetylcholine and MS

Acetylcholine balance is maintained by specific enzymes that have the ability to break down ACh. In one study, patients with relapsing-remitting MS were found to have lower levels of ACh as well as higher activity of ACh-degrading enzymes. This combination creates an imbalanced environment where inflammatory immune cells can escalate. The researchers in this study concluded that the higher levels of degrading enzymes were the primary cause of low ACh levels in MS, rather than a problem with ACh production.[8]

This interdependent relationship between ChAT and AChE is typical of how the body works: Simply put, there are chemicals that create processes, and chemicals that put an end to those processes when appropriate. Above all, our body operates within zones of intricate balance, and it tries to restore that balance as much as possible whenever things go awry. It should be noted here that proper functioning of the acetylcholine system also appears to play a role in remyelination. In animal models of MS, drugs that stop the activity of ChAT (thereby allowing more acetylcholine to be made) also have been shown to improve remyelination.

There are as yet no studies looking specifically at the benefits of choline or phosphatidylcholine for MS. But given how important choline is for acetylcholine and phosphatidylcholine is for the integrity of cellular structure, adding these neurotransmitters in some form to your long-term treatment plan may be beneficial. Furthermore, the gut microbiome produces a significant amount of acetylcholine, so supplementation may well support the gut-brain axis.

Bacopa and Acetylcholine

Bacopa monnieri is an herb that has a long tradition of use as a nerve tonic and memory enhancer, particularly to address the cognitive decline that often comes with aging. Many studies confirm bacopa's ability to enhance memory and cognitive function through a variety of mechanisms. Bacopa appears to modulate the activity of several neurotransmitters, and especially to influence the acetylcholine system by inhibiting AChE and activating ChAT. A few randomized controlled clinical trials with bacopa have shown that it is safe to use and that it improves attention, cognitive processing, and working memory in older adults. As I mentioned earlier, the primary cause of low acetylcholine levels in MS is most likely higher levels of AChE, rather than a problem with neurotransmitter production. Given that bacopa seems to cover all the bases where acetylcholine is concerned, it could be an ideal herb for people with MS to use.

The most abundant neurotransmitter in the body, acetylcholine (ACh) acts both as an excitatory and inhibitory neurotransmitter in the nervous system. It encourages the formation of synapses during fetal development and is responsible for nerve growth and cell proliferation. Research has revealed that to some degree ACh may also be produced by other cells such as immune cells and cells from the endothelium—the inner layer of cells in blood vessels.

Acetylcholine synthesis requires the nutrient choline, which is found predominantly in eggs, meat, nuts, and dairy. People with Alzheimer's disease have low levels of acetylcholine because they have low levels of choline acetyltransferase, the enzyme that converts choline into acetylcholine in the brain,[9] or high levels of acetylcholinesterase, which breaks down acetylcholine.

Our bodies also use choline to make phosphatidylcholine, which is required to support the structural integrity of cell membranes, and sphingomyelin, which is necessary for the production of the myelin sheath.

Given these effects, could consuming higher levels of phosphatidyl-choline or choline slow down the progression of dementia in people with Alzheimer's disease, and be helpful to people with other neurological disorders? A few studies have shown better cognitive performance in adults who both consume higher levels of choline and have higher concentrations of choline in their blood. People who had low choline blood levels also had poorer mental processing speed, integration of physical movement, and executive function than those whose choline concentrations were higher than 8.4 mcmol/L.[10] Another study of more than 1,300 adults aged 36 to 83 years found that those with higher choline intakes had better verbal memory and visual memory.[11]

A few small randomized controlled studies have shown that choline supplements improve cognitive performance in adults.[12] However, a 2015 systematic review of 13 studies on the relationship between choline levels and neurological outcomes in healthy adults found that choline supplements did not result in clear improvements in cognition.[13] This may simply mean choline is not effective in people who do not have cognitive deficits, but it's hard to say.

It is also likely that the *form* of choline used for supplementation is a factor in its effectiveness. This is an issue that plagues the interpretation of results in natural medicine research in general. The same natural substance often comes in a variety of forms, and each form may have varying degrees of bioavailability (a measure of how well the body can absorb and use a nutrient after it's consumed). For example, a 2003 Cochrane review of 12 randomized trials in 265 patients with Alzheimer's disease, 21 with Parkinsonian dementia, and 90 with self-identified memory problems found no clear clinical benefits for Alzheimer's or Parkinsonian dementia for supplementing with lecithin, which contains in the range of 10 to 20 percent phosphatidylcho-line.[14] And there is some evidence to suggest that choline taken in the form of citicoline (a naturally occurring compound commonly found in over-the-counter supplements for brain support) is better utilized by the body.

In short, more studies are needed to clarify the relationship between choline intake and cognitive function, and to determine whether choline supplements might benefit people with Alzheimer's disease or other neurological disorders such as MS.

Medications That Affect Acetylcholine

Many of the drugs prescribed to people with MS have what is called anticholinergic activity. They work, in part, by blocking acetylcholine, which means they can cause confusion and memory problems as side effects. Drugs that have anticholinergic effects include tricyclic antidepressants like amitriptyline (Elavil). Tricyclic antidepressants are prescribed only to younger people precisely because the anticholinergic effects are stronger in older people. In comparison, the SSRI antidepressants are considered to have relatively low anticholinergic activity, but they do have some. SSRIs include citalopram (Celexa), sertraline (Zoloft), and duloxetine (Cymbalta). Antidepressants with the lowest anticholinergic activity are venlafaxine (Effexor) and bupropion (Wellbutrin). Another drug, oxybutynin (Ditropan), which is commonly prescribed to treat MS bladder symptoms, also has anticholinergic effects, as do over-the-counter first-generation antihistamines such as diphenhydramine (Benadryl). I tried oxybutynin, and after I took my first dose, I enjoyed a full night's sleep with no need to get up to urinate—for the first time in many years. However, the following week I began to experience the side effects: constipation, fatigue, and so much mental confusion I couldn't even figure out how to use my coffee grinder in the morning.

If you are on anticholinergic medication, ask your physician about switching to an alternative that doesn't have those effects. It is always good to stay informed about the medications you take, because their side effects may not be fully understood for years after they are put on the market. For example, recent research has established a link between drugs commonly taken for improved sleep and an increased risk of dementia.

Dopamine

Dopamine, like serotonin, is a neurotransmitter also classified as a hormone. Dopamine is an essential element in the brain-reward system and reward-motivated learning. For example, most drugs that have addictive properties trigger the dopamine system to elicit the reward sensation. The downside of dopamine is that the continuous artificial stimulation that occurs in drug addiction leads to desensitization, which ultimately requires increasingly larger doses to achieve the same effect. Opioids, including heroin and fentanyl, for example, act as a continuous artificial stimulant, which explains why the addict constantly seeks stronger drugs and is at risk for overdosing.[15]

Dopamine also plays a role in sleep, mood, attention, learning, behavior, pain processing, movement, and cognition. Dysfunction in the dopamine system is related to schizophrenia, mood disorders, obsessive compulsive disorder (OCD), autism, attention deficit hyperactivity disorder (ADHD), drug addiction, Parkinson's, and others. Dopamine in excess can lead to mania.

Dopamine is involved with motor functions and can stimulate the release of hormones. It stimulates luteinizing hormone, which can trigger testosterone and progesterone release in men and women, respectively. Dopamine deficiency can therefore cause symptoms related to low sex hormones, such as low libido, erectile dysfunction, muscle wasting, PMS, mood swings, and weight gain. Dopamine also interacts with thyroid hormone and prolactin, a hormone that triggers milk production in females and is also involved in other functions, including regulating metabolism, the immune system, and behavior. Studies have shown that individuals with MS, both female and male, have higher levels of serum prolactin than do healthy controls.[16] (Researchers are still investigating why.) Because dopamine inversely impacts prolactin production, it could potentially be beneficial in treating MS.

Dopamine and Inflammation

Dopamine may interact with the immune system and have an anti-inflammatory effect. There may be "cross-talk" between the immune and nervous systems: Certain immune cells have dopamine receptors, and some immune cells can produce and release dopamine. Although the mechanism is not fully understood, dopamine might positively regulate the specific immune parameters that trigger inflammation and ultimately lead to autoimmune reactions. Animal studies have shown that dopamine levels are reduced in several autoimmune conditions in which inflammation is not in check, such as MS, inflammatory bowel disease, rheumatoid arthritis, and lupus. Furthermore, dopamine-type medications have been shown to have anti-inflammatory properties.[17]

Dopamine can directly or indirectly regulate the immune system in neurodegenerative conditions such as Parkinson's disease and Alzheimer's disease. Some researchers believe that the number of dopamine receptors in the immune cells of patients with neurodegenerative diseases is an accurate marker of the extent of disease progression.

Dopamine and MS

The relationship between MS and dopamine is a complex one that requires much more research to elucidate. In MS it is clear that dopamine plays a role in immune activation, but it also acts as an immune suppressant depending on the conditions. Dopamine has the ability to reduce the autoimmune reaction and be neuroprotective, but studies on relapsing-remitting MS have shown that the dopamine pathways are dysfunctional and fail to regulate neuroinflammation. For this reason, MS patients may have inadequate dopamine, putting them at risk for also developing Parkinson's disease.[18]

Dopamine medications have shown some promising immunomodulating actions in animal studies, but not in clinical trials so far. Some researchers suggest that dopamine medications would be more beneficial when combined with immunomodulating medications for MS, such as interferons.[19]

Fatigue is a prominent symptom of MS, and although multiple theories exist, the reasons why such fatigue occurs aren't yet clear. One possible reason is dopamine imbalance. A study of MS patients' brain imaging showed that particular parts of the brain in which dopamine neurons are concentrated were abnormal or damaged. This damage is possibly caused by the autoimmune reactivity associated with MS. Other conditions that damage those parts of the brain, such as traumatic brain injury, are also associated with significant symptoms of fatigue.[20]

Modafinil (Provigil) is an anti-drowsiness drug formulated for use by the US Army, so combat soldiers could fight longer hours. It is also used to treat drowsiness caused by sleep disorders or shift work. It stimulates dopamine production and thus helps people stay alert. It is highly effective in treating MS-related problems with cognitive abilities involving energy, attention, and focus. This drug can be pricey, so insurance companies sometimes prefer cheaper alternatives such as amphetamines, which are neurotoxins and are linked to Parkinson's disease. I tried taking amphetamines at a few dosages, but they didn't help me and I stopped taking them. Then I convinced my neurologist to appeal the insurance company's decision not to pay for modafinil. The appeal was upheld and I was prescribed modafinil. This pill was a game changer in terms of helping with cognitive tasks and maintaining energy. It was an invaluable tool that allowed me to focus when I gave presentations at medical conferences. Five years after I began taking it, fortunately, I discovered that I no longer need it at all, due to a regimen of other treatments that have decreased inflammation.

One big way in which modafinil helped me was in my ability to focus, particularly in social situations. As I described earlier in the book, for people with MS, being in a room in which more than one person is talking can feel like trying to listen to many radio stations playing at once—a nonsensical mélange of competing sound waves. Modafinil helped me screen out the background noise and focus on a single conversation.

To avoid disrupting normal sleep patterns, it's best to take stimulants like modafinil when you first wake up. Alternatively, if you need more energy toward evening, you could break up individual pills into four pieces, and space out taking those quarter-pieces throughout the day. However, taking more than 50 mg after the noon hour can easily cause insomnia. Sometimes it's worth the insomnia, which can also be alleviated by taking melatonin or high doses of an herb called kava (*Piper methysticum*) before going to bed. I do not advise taking stimulants on a regular basis, but stimulants can be an important tool in your MS tool kit.

Mucuna pruriens is an herbal remedy that increases dopamine and can serve as a very mild alternative to modafinil. Although mucuna is not as potent as a prescription pharmaceutical, it also doesn't come with modafinil's side effects, such as heart palpitations.

Glutamate and GABA

Glutamate, which is derived from the amino acid glutamic acid, is an abundant excitatory neurotransmitter. A variety of glutamate receptors are important to learning and memory. Excess glutamate is a concern because it can cause excitotoxicity and be neurotoxic. It is linked to Alzheimer's disease, Parkinson's disease, and brain trauma.[21]

Glutamate is the precursor of GABA, the primary inhibitory neurotransmitter. GABA opposes the actions of the excitatory neurotransmitters, including glutamate. GABA can be neuroprotective and can prevent neurodegeneration caused by excitatory neurotransmitters. One of the proposed causes of beta-amyloid plaque in AD is an imbalance between excitatory and inhibitory neurotransmitters. This imbalance may also underlie early AD cognitive dysfunction.[22]

At least one study has indicated that GABA levels are decreased in the brain of patients with progressive MS. In this study, patients with MS showed reduced motor skills, sensory skills, and verbal memory, as well as slower processing speed. Lower GABA levels corresponded to worse performance. Because GABA is neuroprotective, having very low levels may contribute to worsening neurodegeneration. Therefore, GABA levels may be a marker of disease progression. Research indicates that taking GABA as a supplement could help slow disease progression. Side effects such as lethargy can occur,[23] though I have never seen this in myself or my patients. Kava helps increase GABA levels in the body, and I find it helpful for many of the symptoms related to MS including bladder spasms, laryngospasms, and muscle tension. Kava works quickly; usually 150 mg of kavalactones—a class of lactone compounds found in kava shrubs and commonly used in supplements—produces a response with an hour. If taken before bed, kava can be helpful with sleep and can decrease the incidence of waking up at night due to painful muscle spasms and frequent urination.

———

Despite science's understanding of individual biochemical factors in neurodegeneration, for the most part there are no simple cures. Most likely this is because the causes of neurodegeneration are multifactorial and can't be resolved within a single magic-bullet solution. Early intervention and prevention continue to be our best hope.

CHAPTER 9

Managing MS Day-to-Day

The specific treatment approaches—herbs, hormones, and pharmaceuticals—discussed in earlier chapters of this book all play important roles in addressing some of the physical and emotional symptoms of MS. But I also employ other strategies and complementary therapies that have proven to be effective as I navigate the daily challenges of living with this disease. Throughout my own personal journey, I have found these to be exceptionally important. Some were among my first lines of defense against the unknown, and remain so today.

Not all of these techniques will work for everyone, of course, so I offer them as a sort of menu in this chapter, with anecdotes to illustrate their practicality in my particular circumstance. It's also critical to remember that every day is different—just as every person with MS is different. In a sense, this entire chapter is my personal prescription for living life to the fullest with multiple sclerosis.

Diet

Because I've talked extensively about diet elsewhere in the book, I won't repeat that discussion here. That said, my daily diet is one of the primary tools I use to manage symptoms, so here's a quick summary of my diet-related advice to help promote good brain health:

- Include a variety of healthy fats, including fish, chia, flaxseed, and coconut oils, avocados, and omega-3s.

- Avoid meats that contain added antibiotics or hormones. Choose organic, grass-fed meats whenever possible. Minimize intake of foods that contain added sugar, and don't eat any foods that contain high-fructose corn syrup.
- Stick to a whole-foods-based diet with as many organic foods as possible.

Detoxification

In chapter 2 I discussed the many environmental toxins we're exposed to on an almost daily basis, and the importance of minimizing those exposures in order to protect brain health. Sometimes, though, even that's not enough. That's why I regularly practice—and advise—detoxification, which is a simple process once you know the basics.

Many of the actions you can take to help minimize the effects of toxins work to support the liver, which is responsible for breaking down toxins. Unlike many organic compounds we ingest, environmental toxins that enter the body are fat-soluble, not water-soluble, which makes them difficult to eliminate. The liver must then work hard to convert these chemicals into water-soluble form so they can be excreted in the urine and bile. Without getting too deeply into the complex biochemistry of it, in Phase One detoxification, the liver

Quick Tips to Limit Toxins

- Eat foods grown from certified organic farms.
- Read every food label. Avoid those with chemical additives.
- Choose natural health and beauty products when possible.
- Store food and water in glass containers.
- If you must use a microwave, don't reheat food on or in plastic.
- Avoid Styrofoam completely.

turns harmful substances into less harmful ones via the processes of oxidation, reduction, and hydrolysis. Ironically, this sometimes produces free radicals that, if not removed in Phase Two, can themselves be harmful. In Phase Two (known as the conjugation pathway), the liver adds a molecule or molecules to the substances resulting from Phase One to make them water-soluble.

The liver uses up nutrients in this process, including antioxidants such as vitamin C, alpha-lipoic acid, B vitamins, and amino acids, which makes them all good candidates as detox support supplements.

The supplement called reduced glutathione is an important cofactor of antioxidant enzymes that help recycle antioxidants back to their active state, providing a steady supply to the body. It's known as the master antioxidant and is an important ingredient in the detoxification pathway. Glutathione is a medically proven detoxifier. In hospital emergency rooms, for example, it's given intravenously to protect the livers of patients who overdose on acetaminophen.

Lifestyle and Life Strategies

I find that some of the best strategies I can use to mitigate my symptoms—and, often, the emotions surrounding them—involve making adjustments to how I'm living and going about my days.

These adjustments aren't always easy; nothing is with MS! But I'm fortunate to have Sarika's support. If you have friends and family you can recruit as teammates to help you succeed in making positive lifestyle changes, it can really make a difference. I also know of some people who work with wellness coaches. No matter the approach you take, here are my top recommendations for making your own lifestyle adjustments.

Energy Conservation and Time Management

To be effective at decision making, I need to conserve my energy so that it's available when I need to make important decisions. This first means getting adequate sleep, which in the case of someone with MS might mean napping during the day as well as sleeping at night. In addition, I'm mindful about things like screen time and the amount of time I spend in other types of intense concentration. Taking occasional short breaks allows our brains some refresh time, which overall contributes to better cognitive function.

Another successful strategy I use to conserve energy is to limit my involvement in situations and relationships that aren't positive, and saying no to social invitations when I know I need the rest. For some people, this can be difficult. After all, we all want to nourish our relationships and have fun. And sometimes people may be offended when we turn down their invitations. You don't even need to bring MS into the discussion—unless you want to. Just explain simply and politely that you need to take some time to recharge. Those who accept this will be glad to socialize with you another time. Those who don't are people you may wish to avoid anyway.

Attitude Adjustment

If you or a loved one has struggled with MS-related memory issues, you know how discouraging it can be, and how alone you can feel. By sharing what I've learned, I hope to reassure you that it is indeed possible to reduce the impacts of memory impairment in ways that help you regain your sense of control.

When I first learned of my diagnosis and began living "officially" as an MS patient, I often felt disappointed about my situation. Deflated about it being so much work to tie my shoes. Disappointed that going to the gym was mentally challenging because I had to sequence all the steps of getting undressed and then dressed in the locker room, and recognizing which was the proper footwear to put on when. And confused that—despite my best efforts rarely I couldn't "use my words," as we parents tell our children.

Earlier in the book, I mentioned how MS is like surfing. Rather than let setbacks like these repeatedly slam my emotions into the deepest depths, I chose to ride them out. But if you can practice a little detachment and attitude adjustment as part of your medicine, you may be surprised at the positive results!

Organization and Systems

A 2014 study of people with MS showed that keeping your home organized and avoiding clutter can have a big positive effect.[1] Participants who used a

Learning Not to Be Defeated

The reason babies are unable to hold their heads up is because their myelin sheaths haven't fully developed. Ironically, at the time in my life when my kids' myelin was developing, mine was breaking down . . . leading us, in many ways, to the same exact place physically.

While observing my two toddlers one day, it hit me: *I had more things in common with them that I might think!* In all their goofy clumsiness, in all the things they were striving to learn to do, I was right there, too. Just because there was a 40-year age difference between us didn't mean we couldn't learn many of the same things at the same time, right?

I never thought that in my 40s I'd be learning how to tie my shoes with clumsy fingers, practicing vowel sounds while taking speech lessons, and working on organizing the sequential process of something as seemingly simple as getting dressed. I'm thankful my kids were there to show me how excited they were whenever they mastered a new skill. That's when I realized that just because I'm having to relearn basic skills I mastered 30 years ago, it doesn't have to be a depressing experience. Knowing that I'm trying my best is empowering itself.

protocol developed to help them stay organized had a sense of accomplishment in controlling their environment, reported fewer falls, felt less isolated, increased their ability to find their medications, felt a better general sense of cognitive clarity during activities of daily living (ADLs), and established a sense of accomplishment in controlling their environments.

Every day we need to perform any number of cognitive tasks, including picking out clothes and getting dressed, doing whatever we do to make a living, caring for our children, cooking, cleaning, and pursuing our hobbies and interests. Even when I'm feeling my best, these tasks can take a lot of mental energy. One way I make things easier on myself is to ensure I'm organized and have systems in place that streamline things as much as possible. Here are some strategies that might work for you:

A place for everything, everything in its place. Getting dressed is harder if your dresser drawers and closet aren't organized. Doing home repairs is harder if you can't find your tools. Save time and stress by developing systematized storage for everything from clothes to sporting goods, tools to pantry staples.

Plan chores in advance. Plan errands and household tasks in advance. Instead of being forced to go shopping or do laundry when desperation arises, make a chore schedule for shopping, laundry, and other common tasks. You'll find yourself in fewer "emergency" situations. And when you are feeling challenged by symptoms, you can shift a planned chore to a better time.

Rely on your calendar. Calendars are a must for scheduling events and appointments of all sorts, from doctor visits to birthdays, work deadlines to social events. Even when my symptoms are minimal, I don't know where I'd be without mine. Calendars don't need to be fancy. Use what works for you, whether it's a traditional paper datebook or a slick mobile app. And get in the habit of checking it regularly.

Use list power. Remembering items for a grocery list, chores that need doing at home or work, or bills that need paying can be challenging for anyone. Couple that with the cognitive symptoms of MS, and things can quickly become overwhelming. To avoid this, use the power of lists. Make them on paper, type them into notes on your phone or computer, or even use a mobile app.

Stick on some labels. When my symptoms were at their worst, Sarika labeled bowls, plates, and cups in the kitchen by size, because it was very exhausting for me to determine the difference among sizes. That simple task felt as challenging as playing an advanced game of 3-D chess. Labeling can be very helpful in less extreme circumstances as well. Label drawers in kitchens, bedrooms, and bathrooms to identify their contents. Labels in the workshop, in the garage, and on storage bins for sports or hobby gear can be helpful, too. I use a mechanical label machine, which is commonly available at office supply stores.

Meditation

Research shows that meditation is a powerful tool for increasing attention, regulating emotion, improving psychological balance, increasing self-awareness, and enhancing overall health and well-being. It is also particularly effective in reducing the stress associated with chronic disease—which is doubly important considering the implications of stress on cognitive health. Numerous studies have linked stress with declines in neuroplasticity, memory, and the ability to learn and retain information, for example. For these reasons alone, stress-management strategies should be at the top of every MS patient's daily task list.

I started meditating while studying in India during my college years. Since then I have attended vipassana meditation retreats that include 10 days of silence and a full schedule of meditation from early morning until past nightfall. Meditation helps me to be less reactive; I am better able to calmly observe physical sensations such as pain and to decrease my reaction to them. Despite experiencing quite intense pain related to MS, I never take painkillers, and thus I have avoided possible side effects including habituation and addiction. And meditation retreats have done more than increase my ability to accept and tolerate my symptoms. In fact, I met Sarika at a vipassana meditation center!

Exercise

Aerobic exercise shows many beneficial effects on cognitive function and well-being.[2] According to the findings of a 2018 study led by a researcher from the Department of Movement Sciences and Wellbeing at Parthenope University of Naples in Naples, Italy, in collaboration with colleagues from a variety of institutions throughout the country, exercise increased gray matter in the frontal and hippocampal regions, increased levels of neurotrophic factors, increased blood flow to the brain, increased academic achievement, improved learning and memory, and prevented cognitive decline and the risk of dementia. In addition, exercise has effects on mental health, including reducing depression, anxiety, and tension and increasing confidence, emotional stability, and sexual satisfaction. Exercise may contribute to improving memory, and part of that influence is via the endocrine system. Some studies indicate that exercise can help balance the hypothalamic-pituitary-adrenal (HPA) axis, although it doesn't necessarily reduce cortisol levels.[3] High-intensity exercise also has been shown to increase or balance testosterone levels.[4] And animal studies show that regular exercise can improve thyroid hormone levels and spatial learning.[5] This is important because, as we saw in chapter 7, maintaining hormonal balance is critical in MS, because of both the positive and negative impacts hormones can exert in the brain and CNS.

To keep my brain and spirit fit, I exercise regularly. I ski, hike with my family, and walk to work when I can. Remember, you don't have to climb Mount Everest or run a marathon to get the benefits of exercise. Studies show you can get benefits from physical activity in as little as 30 minutes per day.

My goal is to exercise as much as I can when I can. During periods of exacerbation I limit myself to gentle yoga. During relatively good times, I aim to exercise a minimum of twice a week. This can be in the form of gentle walking or, on great days, skiing or biking.

I find yoga helpful for alleviating the discomfort of muscle spasms and general muscle tightness. But I do cardiovascular workouts such as running whenever I can. After some cardio, I always feel better. My mind feels more awake, and positive emotions increase when I exercise. At the time of this writing, I'm able to do cardio exercises like running/skiing about half the days of the year; the other half, I'm usually not able to because of issues related to autonomic dysfunction or general weakness.

Like me, many people with MS have experienced periods of fatigue, muscle spasms, and paralysis that, at least in the moment, make exercise difficult, if not impossible. But if you do your best to incorporate regular exercise into your life when it is possible, you will likely experience many benefits. Studies have shown that exercise, ranging from walking and yoga to resistance training and aerobic workouts, can reduce fatigue; improve gait, muscle endurance, and other aspects of functional activity; reduce depression and stress; and improve subjective well-being and mood.[6]

Before you begin your own exercise program:

Consult with your health care provider if you have significant physical limitations. **Start slowly.** In exercise, as in all types of care, the rule is "first, do no harm."
     If you leap into exercise with too much enthusiasm, you could well end up with an injury that would have a net negative impact. It doesn't take herculean effort to increase your strength level, improve your balance, and enhance your mood. So remember, it's not about being an "iron person," but about attaining a level of fitness that enriches your life. Go easy, especially at the start, and the rewards will come in time.

Schedule a time, and be consistent. We all live busy lives, and many of us have schedules that are heavily booked. Because of this, it's important to set aside a dedicated exercise time. A few times a week should be the minimum, and you can exercise every day if you have the time and inclination. But if you want to achieve a higher fitness level, consistency should be your goal.

Focus on stretching, resistance, and aerobics. As mentioned above, research shows that stretching (including yoga), resistance training (such as weight lifting and bodyweight exercises), and aerobics bring a range of benefits to people with MS.

Include some variety. Choosing a variety of fitness options provides two main benefits. First, it ensures that you'll be exercising as many body systems as possible, from the heart and lungs to large muscle groups and joints, ligaments, and tendons. Second, it can help to stave off boredom—the kind of boredom that makes you stop exercising. If you want to cycle one day, garden the next, and hit a yoga class on another day and it works for you, by all means do it! But if the same routine every day keeps you going, that's okay, too. It's your body and your choice.

Sleep

For all people, sleep plays a critical role in physical and mental health. A restorative sleep gives the body and the mind a chance to rest, repair, recharge, and prepare for the challenges of the day ahead. But when someone doesn't get a good night's sleep, the next day can be—well—a nightmare. It's harder to concentrate and harder to think. Your supply of patience quickly drains, and the ability to problem-solve drops. For people with chronic sleep issues, these problems are compounded.

Unfortunately, people with MS are more likely than the general population to experience a hard time getting a good night's sleep. The causes of these sleep issues are many. Here are some of the most common:

- Insomnia
- Restless leg syndrome
- Nocturnal leg spasms
- Frequent need to urinate

- Narcolepsy
- Sleep apnea
- Stress
- Depression

During episodes when I'm not well, I might need to get up as many as eight times a night, mostly to manage autonomic symptoms such as thermoregulation issues (getting too hot or sweating profusely), blood pressure and pulse issues related to autonomic dysreflexia, and choking on saliva. (In chapter 10 I explain what autonomic dysreflexia is all about.)

If you experience sleep issues, it can be hard to get the rest you need. To get help, consult with your health care provider. Some people with MS don't have any diagnosed sleep condition, but even they need to pay special attention to their sleep habits. A lack of sleep can exacerbate many of the symptoms of MS and can even extend their duration. When it comes to achieving restful sleep, the following tips can help.

Create and follow a regular bedtime routine. Depending upon your personal preferences, you might set aside a time shortly before bed to bathe, do some yoga or meditation, or read a book. Avoid emotional conversations and stimulating media during this time.

Exercise regularly. Aerobic exercise causes you to release endorphins, which can promote sound sleep. As little as 30 minutes of moderate aerobic exercise can have a positive impact.[7]

Don't use your bedroom as a hangout spot. Give your body and mind the message: The bed is for sleeping.

Make good dietary choices. Avoid heavy meals, caffeine, alcohol, and other nonmedical drugs before bedtime.

Avoid screens. A number of studies have shown that computer, TV, tablet, and smartphone screens can disrupt normal sleep patterns. Avoid screens in the two to three hours before bedtime, and keep them out of the bedroom completely.[8]

Create a comfortable sleeping space. Keep your room cool, dark, and quiet. Make sure your mattress, pillows, and bed linens are clean and comfortable. And again, keep screens *out* of the bedroom.

Supplements and Herbal Remedies

In addition to melatonin, natural medicine offers many herbs known as nervines. These botanicals are helpful allies for improving sleep and soothing the nervous system. Three of my favorite herbs in that regard are valerian, hops, and passionflower. None of these herbs dull mental concentration or carry the risk of dependency.

Melatonin

As discussed in chapter 7, melatonin is responsible for regulating the sleep-wake cycle.

We know that melatonin levels in the blood start to rise at night when it's dark, and are suppressed during the day by light. Exposure to light at night (including from computer screens and other electronic devices) can block melatonin production. There is some evidence that supplementing with melatonin is helpful for sleep conditions such as delayed sleep phase syndrome. Melatonin may also provide some relief from chronic insomnia and the symptoms of jet lag. I take 3 to 6 mg before bed on nights I need it. Most of the year I don't need it, unless I have taken pharmaceuticals (such as steroids) to manage my MS symptoms.

Valerian

The root of the plant *Valeriana officinalis*, or valerian, has a long history of use for sleep problems and anxiety. It has also been the subject of a great deal of research. Studies show that valerian can help with falling asleep more quickly as well as improving the quality and amount of sleep. Valerenic acid, one of the many bioactive compounds found in valerian, has been shown to enhance levels of the neurotransmitter GABA by inhibiting its breakdown. GABA helps create a sense of calm and relaxation in the nervous system. (By the way, prescription anti-anxiety medications exert their effect via the same mechanism as valerian—inhibiting the breakdown of GABA.) Low levels of GABA are associated with poor-quality sleep and anxiety. Healthy levels are required for deep and restorative sleep, particularly the stages of slow-wave and REM sleep. Valerian also has antispasmodic properties, meaning it helps to relax tense or cramping muscles. In some people, valerian can act paradoxically and have a stimulating effect. Be on the lookout for that, and either stop taking it or decrease the dosage or frequency if you suspect it's having that effect on you.

Hops

Hops (*Humulus lupulus*) is a member of the hemp family, and is well known as an ingredient in beer. Like valerian, hops support healthy levels of GABA in the nervous system. In addition, it may obtain its sleep-inducing effects through the same hormone mechanism as melatonin. Hops helps lower core body temperature, which is an important step in how the body prepares physiologically for sleep. Hops is faster acting than valerian—which becomes more effective over a period of days—and thus hops is often used in combination with valerian and is more effective for promoting sleep when used in that pairing. Hops also has antioxidant and anti-inflammatory activity.

Passionflower

Passiflora incarnata is the species of passionflower that supports restorative sleep and soothes the nervous system. *Passiflora* increases levels of GABA. Like valerian, passionflower has antispasmodic properties and can help relieve muscle spasms.

Thermoregulation

Heat can exacerbate MS symptoms because it can reduce the already lessened ability of demyelinated nerves to carry signals throughout the body. In addition, sweat glands, which help to cool the body in warm temperatures, may function less effectively in people with MS. As a result, everything from thought processes to gait, speech, and other muscular movements can be impaired.[9]

According to a 2010 study, somewhere between 60 and 80 percent of those living with MS notice a temporary worsening of their clinical signs and neurological symptoms when it's hot out or they're otherwise exposed to heat. Known as Uhthoff's syndrome, this negative effect of heat on MS symptoms was first documented in 1890 by Wilhelm Uhthoff, a German ophthalmologist who noticed that MS patients with optic neuritis experienced poorer vision when they exercised. Later, clinicians discovered that it was not the exercise, but the increase in body temperature, that caused the poor vision, as well as an increase in other MS-related symptoms including fatigue and motor difficulty.

For some people with MS, heat can cause severe symptoms, including not being able to walk and/or talk in hot weather. In fact, many physicians used to employ a hot bath as an MS diagnostic tool. If a patient placed in a warm bath experienced neurological symptoms, MS would be considered as a diagnosis.

The good news is that the effects on MS symptoms produced by heat are temporary and will usually decrease once the body cools down. However, it's important for people with Uhthoff's syndrome to avoid overheating whenever possible. Keep an eye on outdoor temperatures, and use air-conditioning to maintain comfortable indoor temperatures. If you must go out when it's warm, stick to shady spaces whenever possible. Use cool drinks, a hat, a parasol, or cooling gear such as ice packs and headbands to keep your body temperature lower.

In addition, make sure that friends and family know about your susceptibility to heat so they can provide aid when you need it. And if you are feeling stressed from heat, get to a cool space as soon as possible, treat yourself with cool drinks, compresses, or ice packs, and call emergency medical support if necessary. Hospital emergency rooms are equipped with cooling suits to treat MS patients disabled by heat.

However, it's important to also recognize that cold temperatures can worsen symptoms of people with MS. Such people may experience increased pain, spasticity, cramping, and muscle stiffness when exposed to cold. To prevent and alleviate difficulties with cold, plan ahead. Dress in layers that can be added or removed according to fluctuations in temperature. Adjust indoor temperatures by adjusting the thermostat or turning on space heaters, and adjust your clothing or cover up with a blanket to help prevent getting a chill. When necessary, use hot beverages to warm yourself from the inside (but keep in mind the possible effect of caffeinated beverages on sleep and energy levels). Your health care practitioner may also prescribe medications that can help you deal with cold-related muscle issues and pain.

Stress Management

Dealing with the symptoms and challenges of MS can exacerbate stress—which, in turn, can exacerbate symptoms. It's a frustrating loop that in itself impacts quality of life. One thing I want to mention here—and I'm adamant about this—is that it's important not to blame patients for their MS. While anxiety and stress can clearly *result* from MS, studies show that they don't *cause* it. Misdirected blame only makes them feel worse. People with MS have long reported that stress seemed to make their MS symptoms worse.

That said, avoiding stress altogether is unrealistic, so managing it is the most practical approach. Stress reduction through physical activity and mindfulness-based activities has been shown to help lower excessive cortisol levels.

One clinical trial tested a "mindfulness-based stress reduction program" for older adults with cognitive problems or anxiety. The program involved teaching the participants how to meditate and do yoga. The participants continued practicing for three to six months, and then their progress was tested. As compared with a control group, participants in the program showed significant improvement in their memories and depression and anxiety levels.[10]

Managing MS can be a difficult and time-consuming task. Depending upon the individual, there can be an overwhelming number of symptoms, along with a similar or greater number of strategies for minimizing or delaying them. There may be a variety of appointments to track and attend, from neurology and physical therapy to massage and vocational, optical, and nutritional therapies. Patients may be pursuing any number of strategies for managing MS, from taking IV infusions and daily physical therapy regimens to occupational therapy appointments and daily urinary catheterizations.

At the same time, life goes on. There are jobs and relationships, social and school events. There is the need to parent children and take care of older family members, too. And flare-ups of MS symptoms can make it harder to meet these obligations, thus making stress worse.

One MS study showed something remarkable: that a reduction in stress could help slow the growth of MS-related brain lesions.[11] This study, which focused on patients with relapsing MS at three sites in the United States, used a standardized stress reduction treatment called stress management therapy for multiple sclerosis, or SMT-MS. The strategies used to reduce stress included "teaching problem solving skills, relaxation, increasing positive activities, cognitive restructuring, and enhancement of social support."[12]

Given the stresses inherent with managing MS (and in managing life in general!), as well as the documented positive effects of stress reduction, it's important for people with MS to do what they can to minimize stress and its impact on their lives. Depending upon your needs and interests, your stress reduction plan could include many of the subjects covered in this chapter, such as exercise, meditation, avoiding stressful situations, getting sufficient sleep, spending time with friends and family, working with a therapist, practicing assertiveness, listening to music, and spending time being creative.

My personal habits include focusing on life versus my illness and setting boundaries to focus on my wellness. This includes keeping my medical appointments to no more than three hours a week on two days a week, as well as having an hour a day to focus on taking all of my medicines and herbs, and completing any related tasks such as reordering them when I need to. I also try to go with the flow, and remind myself that my "new normal" means that I can't maintain the same highly active life that I did before MS.

Relationships

When it comes to relationships, all of us work to find a balance. We want to develop rich and rewarding relationships with friends and family. But often, that means making choices and setting boundaries that allow us to maintain a comfortable personal space. And for people with MS, their friends, and their families, it's particularly important to nourish relationships and set appropriate boundaries.

Fortunately, my family and friends all have done an outstanding job supporting and caring for me and recognizing my limits, while also empowering me to make my own decisions about what I am able to do.

MS can have both small and large impacts on the way we engage with people around us. MS may lessen the amount of energy people can devote to relationships. And it may reduce their ability to participate in social activities. The challenges of dealing with symptoms of MS or caring for a loved one with the disease can put stress on even strong connections, causing the growth of guilt, anger, and resentment. One recent study has shown that MS brain lesions can reduce people's ability to interpret social and emotional cues, making communication harder.[13] For me, during exacerbations it becomes difficult to recognize people outside my immediate family and a few close friends. When I go into town on such days, most guys between the age of about 20 and 50 all look like the same person to me. So when a person waves at me, I'm not always sure which friend it is, because everyone looks like my friend—which is actually a pleasant thing as long as I'm not feeling self-conscious.

Given these difficulties, how can someone with MS maintain healthy, rich relationships with the people they care about? In my experience, the pathway contains four steps: education, boundary setting, delegation, and honest communication.

Education

As I described earlier in the book, for the person with MS and those around them, the initial diagnosis often brings a measure of both relief (*Oh! That's why these strange things have been happening!*) and anxiety (*Oh no! What do we do now?*). The world suddenly becomes more complicated. There's a complex and mysterious disease to learn about, understand, and learn to live with. What was once the daily routine of life may now be impossible to sustain. There will be adjustments to schedules and eating habits, sleep patterns, and mobility. All this can be baffling and hard to cope with. But education makes things easier for everyone. Here's what you can do to educate yourself (and others) about MS.

Ask your health care provider for basic information and reliable sources. Books, magazines, and the internet offer a wealth of information about MS, but not all of it is accurate. Your caregiver can likely provide you with some basic information about MS and your treatment options. And at the end of this book, I've included a set of answers to frequently asked questions that offers a lot of good info. But if you want to go deeper (and you probably should), your caregiver can point you to reliable resources with more in-depth information, including links to support groups and databases of MS information. *Encourage friends and family to learn more.* Many of the stresses related to an MS diagnosis occur due to interactions with well-intentioned but uninformed family members and friends. Such folks may, for example, suggest unproven "miracle" treatments or blame a person with MS for failing to participate in family and social events. Once they learn the basics about MS, many of these situations can be avoided. My favorite documentary about MS is called *When I Walk.* It's made by Jason DaSilva, who was diagnosed with primary progressive MS while in his 20s. It explains well what it can feel like to have MS.

Consider your audience. Not everyone is capable of understanding complicated information about the MS diagnosis, its effects on the individual, and the treatment plan. Young children are one example of a group for whom the information presented should be limited and relatively simple. They might be told, for example, that their parent is sick and that the disease they have might mean they have to sleep more, use a cane, or eat different foods. But the children would not need to know as much about the situation as a closely related adult would. It's a good idea to adjust the information you give out to people depending upon their level of understanding of medicine. For example, my children often think that some things that I have a hard time doing, such as putting together a puzzle with them, picking up the right toothbrush, or finding the right clothes for them, are simply Papa being silly. Focusing on the fact that I have a brain disease would be difficult for them.

One challenge for me during exacerbations is understanding social norms, and remembering what is appropriate to say and to whom. Even more challenging is recognizing emotional cues from others.

Boundaries

Boundaries help all of us negotiate life on our own terms. We define our relationships by the boundaries we set, and clear boundaries can help us to manage expectations and avoid misunderstandings and hard feelings. All people have a right to decide what activities and events are right for them. Be assertive about self-care and getting the rest, exercise, downtime, and nutrition you need to feel as good as you can.

Communication

It's often been said that communication is a two-way street, and that's true. But it's also a responsibility. You can't control what anyone else chooses to communicate about themselves, you, or your MS. But you can clearly and assertively communicate your needs and your expectations for any relationship. Choosing to stay silent may help you avoid a few uncomfortable moments, but it can cost you years of anguish. Only the person experiencing MS knows exactly how it feels and what their needs are. When you don't clearly communicate your needs and expectations, you're asking others to guess them. And that's a recipe for hard times and hurt feelings.

Dating and Sex

MS can affect both the physical and the emotional aspects of romantic relationships. Damage to the nervous system can reduce a person's ability to become sexually aroused. Men may have difficulty achieving erection or ejaculating. Women may experience reduced sensation in the clitoral or vaginal area, painful sensitivity, or vaginal dryness. Fatigue and muscle spasticity may also reduce interest in sexual activity or make it more difficult. And men and women may experience urinary leakage during intercourse. The impact of these issues can cause emotional responses including lower self-esteem, anger, anxiety, and depression.[14]

That said, many people with MS have pleasurable and fulfilling sex lives. What's the best way to make this happen? First, educate yourself about sexual issues and MS. And if sexual issues become a problem, speak up! Talk to your care provider. They may be able to provide medication that can help, or offer suggestions for restorative approaches to sexual and emotional issues. Talk therapy and meditation may help reduce the emotional impact. One of the most important ways to minimize difficulties with sexual issues and MS is effective communication between partners.

When MS is a factor in a romantic relationship, it's time to dial up the communication meter. Make sure both partners understand the possible impact of MS on the sexual relationship. Vitality and sexual desire often reinforce each other. In many instances, just being able to sleep well and exercise are the best way to allow your body to experience and enjoy being sexually aroused.

Women's Issues and MS

Women are about four times more likely than men to be diagnosed with MS. Hormones likely play a role in this difference, but researchers don't have a clear picture of all the reasons. Beyond diagnosis, many women have gender-related questions and concerns about their disease.

Pregnancy

For women of reproductive age, some of the most common questions concern pregnancy. Long ago, physicians advised women that pregnancy would make their MS symptoms worse, and that MS could negatively affect the fetus or increase the number of complications in the pregnancy. The good news is that we now know that none of these concerns are valid. Women often experience a lessening of symptoms of MS during pregnancy. And the rates of pregnancy complications, spontaneous abortions, stillbirths, and genetic defects are the same for women with MS as for women without it. In the postpartum period, many women experience a temporary increase in their MS symptoms or a relapse in MS. However, pregnancy does not seem to have any long-term impact on the progression of MS.[15]

Menstruation and Menopause

Some women have reported increases of MS symptoms during their period and in postmenopause. Again, these effects are likely linked to differing hormone levels. For some women, hormone replacement therapy (HRT) may lessen the symptoms of MS postmenopause (see also the "Estrogen" section of chapter 7 for more about HRT).

Support Groups

If MS is making you or a loved one feel isolated and alone, support groups can help. But for some people, seeing and talking with a group of patients—many of whom may be experiencing far worse symptoms—can be discouraging. At my first support group meeting, I was one of the only people who was able to walk. Some patients were seated in a wheelchair with an attached IV pole. And everyone reported taking from 10 to as many as 20 different drugs, which was intimidating to me.

Still, MS support groups can be of great value. In these groups, people with MS gather to talk about their experiences, build networks of supportive friends, and share information about how to manage their disease effectively and live rich, fulfilling lives. Those who don't live within reach of a group or who are otherwise unable to attend such meetings can join an online support group and communicate via chat or video. Support groups are a great way for people with MS to educate themselves, expand their social networks, and just have fun.

Aging

All human beings face natural challenges due to the aging process. Our muscle tone decreases. Our memories aren't as sharp as they once were. MS can accentuate such problems. According to a study at the University of Illinois at Urbana-Champaign, older adults with MS have decreased balance, gait speed, and lower extremity strength as compared with older adults who do not have MS.[16] And older people with MS may experience a greater incidence of other conditions as well, from pneumonia and bladder problems to cognitive impairment and osteoporosis.[17] On the upside, though, as some people age, their immune systems become less active, and in these cases the MS progression can become quiet on its own.

Given these findings, it's critically important for older people with MS to pay attention to all aspects of their health, to carefully follow their treatment plan, and to report any changes in function to their caregiver as soon as possible, so that adjustments in the care plan can be made. As I age, the main thing I notice is that my first neurologist was right. Overall, my prognosis was good, he said, but he also told me that the effects of aging would impact my disease process and symptoms such that I would notice it as getting worse.

Bladder and Bowel Health

Bladder and bowel issues are common for people with MS. As these complications can make life less pleasant and can lead to long-term health issues, it's best to treat them quickly and effectively. In addition to Western medical treatments for these issues, a number of restorative treatments can help.

Supporting Healthy Bladder Function

Bladder problems such as urinary spasms, urinary frequency, urinary retention, and infections are common in MS. Some patients may need to use diapers and may need to catheterize daily. Other supportive measures can also be helpful for relaxing bladder spasms, helping ease the emptying of the bladder, and dealing with urinary retention. I find several herbs to be helpful, for example, depending on the severity of the bladder tension, bladder spasm, and the pain level experienced.

Kava can be the most helpful herb for severe spasms and pain. Kava root may be used as a tea or, more commonly, as a tincture extract or capsule taken several times a day to reduce ongoing spasm or discomfort or as needed to relieve episodic spasms.

Cramp bark (*Viburnum opulus*) helps relieve mild to moderate bladder spasms, relaxing the bladder and the pelvic area in general. Cramp bark may be used as a tincture dosed at ½ to 1 teaspoon several times a day. It also makes a light, pleasant-tasting tea. Use 1 tablespoon cramp bark to 8 ounces boiling water, steep 5 to 10 minutes, and then strain. Drink the tea while it is warm, one to three times daily. Another bladder-relaxing herb tea can be made from 1 teaspoon each of dried catnip and chamomile. Steep 10 minutes in 16 ounces boiling water and then strain. Drink warm or cool throughout the day.

Hyoscyamine (also known as daturine) is a naturally occurring plant alkaloid that can be dispensed by an herbalist; it's also synthetically available as a prescription. It's used to treat bladder spasms and other lower abdominal disorders including ulcers and irritable bowel syndrome.

Dealing with Urinary Retention

- Avoid foods that can aggravate the bladder, such as red wine, spicy food, and caffeine.
- For urinary retention in men, remaining seated on the toilet for five minutes can help to fully empty the bladder.
- Warm baths, especially in the evening before bed, can help with relieving urinary retention and emptying the bladder. This allows patients to sleep better as it decreases the need to get up frequently throughout the night.
- Herbal teas made from diuretic plants such as parsley, fennel seed, hibiscus, and lemongrass may be used to help the bladder empty with more ease. Try a mix of 1 teaspoon each of hibiscus flower, fennel seed, and lemongrass in a teapot. Cover with 16 ounces boiling water, steep 5 minutes, and strain. Drink as a warm infusion or as an iced tea. Including fresh parsley in salads and sauces also supports bladder emptying.
- Uribel is a prescription medication that includes an antibiotic and an antiseptic to treat urinary infection, an antispasmodic to treat cramps, and a pain reliever similar to aspirin.

Preventing and Treating UTIs

Urinary infections can be a common trigger for MS attacks. New neurological symptoms can remain permanently after the UTI is gone. For this reason, it is important to take measures to prevent UTIs, and it is also essential to treat UTIs *as quickly as possible.*

Preventive measures include increasing fluid intake, particularly water and herbal teas, because dehydration increases the risk of UTI. Adequate daily fluid intake can go a long way as prevention. Adding a probiotic to your daily supplement program will support and strengthen the health of the urinary microbiome.

Consider taking cranberry capsules (500 mg) on a daily basis if you are prone to urinary infections. Cranberry creates an environment in the urinary tract in which microbes can't thrive, thus reducing the incidence of UTI. D-mannose, which is found in cranberries, is also available as a supplement that can be used to keep *E. coli* from attaching to the bladder wall. People often ask whether drinking cranberry juice works. Unsweetened cranberry juice can be helpful, but many people find it too tart to drink regularly.

The following approaches can be helpful both in preventing and treating UTIs:

- My favorite treatment for UTI is buchu (*Agathosma betulina*) essential oil. Put 3 drops in a glass of water and drink, or apply the 3 drops to a small piece of bread and eat. Take twice a day for 10 days.
- Essential oils of herbs such as thyme and oregano act as antiseptics. Since these oils exit the body through the urinary tract, essential teas or tinctures of them can be used to treat UTI. Try taking ½ teaspoon of thyme tincture mixed into 4 ounces of water three to five times a day for 7 to 10 days.
- Other useful herbs for treating UTI include uva ursi (*Arctostaphylos uva-ursi*) as a tea or extract, and berberine—a natural substance found in barberry (*Berberis*)—capsules, taking 200 to 300 mg daily for 7 days. Goldenseal (*Hydrastis canadensis*) is also useful for UTIs because of its high levels of berberine.

Supporting Bowel Health

Peristalsis is a fancy name for the way the things we consume move through our digestive tract. The opposite of peristalsis is *constipation*. Although I didn't immediately suffer from this particular side effect of MS, it descended upon me quite rapidly—and persistently—following a particularly intense MS attack a few years after my diagnosis. Where I once took this basic bodily function for granted, I now struggled to remember what normal elimination felt like.

There are a variety of reasons for constipation among people with MS, but the primary reason is demyelination in the area of the brain responsible for communicating with the bowels. And according to the National Multiple Sclerosis Society, constipation is the most commonly reported digestive complaint among MS patients.[18]

The good news is, unlike so many other effects of this disease, mild constipation can be treated with relative ease. Patients can usually find relief by practicing the same good habits that benefit the general population: hydrating adequately; consuming enough fiber; establishing a daily time to go; avoiding unnecessary stress; and using stool softeners when indicated. And, as explained earlier in the book, restoring and maintaining a healthy microbiome is key to digestive function.

For Mild Constipation

Many foods, including prunes, figs, fresh plums, melons, and pumpkin, have a positive influence on bowel health. Food-based treatments can help with mild constipation. Here are two tasty, simple, and effective recipes for encouraging bowel function.

Prune-flax blend. Flaxseeds are rich in omega oils, making them very soothing to the GI tract. Their fiber provides healthy food for the microbiome. To make this blend, chop 5 prunes into small pieces. Add 1 teaspoon flaxseeds and 1 cup boiling water. Let cool for 10 minutes (the mixture will thicken as it cools). Eat this blend daily: half the mixture in the evening and the other half the following morning (cool or reheated, as you prefer). It should be the first thing and the last thing you consume each day.

Pumpkin-flax purée. Enjoy this purée daily for healthy bowel function. Combine ½ cup puréed pumpkin with ½ teaspoon cinnamon and 1 teaspoon flax oil and mix well. Eat ¼ cup two times a day.

For More Severe Constipation

For more stubborn constipation, you may need to use osmotic laxatives, ones containing magnesium, or stronger drugs like lubiprostone.

As a first step, try taking fiber supplements, osmotic laxatives, or herbal laxatives in the evening. Magnesium taken daily can help to keep the bowel relaxed and less irritable, contributing to regularity and ease of bowel movements.

All of these options act as osmotic laxatives, helping the body absorb water into the gastrointestinal tract. However, in my experience, osmotic diuretics are not that effective when constipation is neurogenic.

The most effective treatment is plants such as cascara (*Rhamnus purshiana*), yellow dock (*Rumex crispus*), and senna (*Cassia senna*). All three of these herbs act as GI stimulants. I usually recommend cascara sagrada or yellow dock root instead of senna. They are less likely to cause tummy discomfort and are still very effective. Cascara extract is traditionally used and non-habit-forming. I suggest taking either of these herbal treatments in tincture extract form diluted in a warm cup of fennel or ginger tea.

Another excellent option is triphala, which has a long tradition of use in Ayurvedic medicine for digestive issues. Triphala is a mixture of three herbs that are native to India: amla (*Emblica officinalis*), bibhitaki (*Terminalia bellerica*), and haritaki (*T. chebula*). It acts as a natural laxative and also soothes gastrointestinal inflammation. Typical doses are between 500 mg and 1 gram a day. I recommend you start at the lower end of the range to see what amount works best for you. Triphala is available in many forms, but I prefer the powder. I usually add it to a cup of warm water and honey. Take it between meals for better absorption.

Glycerin suppositories can also help stimulate a bowel movement.

Given that peristalsis is initiated by healthy serotonin levels, support for serotonin production and function may also reduce constipation. Try using HTP, which is extracted from the seeds of *Griffonia simplicifolia* (an herb native to Ghana). HTP stimulates serotonin, an important neurotransmitter in the enteric nervous system involved in bowel function.

And of course, a strong, bitter cup of black coffee with no added sugar or milk can also help with constipation. Because of its caffeine content, coffee should be used for laxative purposes only in the morning.

Other methods of emptying the bowels include mechanical elimination such herbal enemas and colonic irrigation. In advanced cases of bowel and bladder dysfunction, mechanical emptying is required daily via enemas and catheterization.

Herbal enema is a traditional preparation using water and steeped herbal teas. The soothing local action helps to relax the bowel, releasing tension and spasm, both of which may accompany constipation. Many aromatic garden herbs such as holy basil, lemon balm, catnip, and mint may be used for the relaxing, soothing action they have on the large intestine and colon.

I recommend using herbal enemas monthly; at a minimum once every three months. This acts to tone the bowel, establish regular bowel movements, and clean toxics out of the bowels. Getting rid of the garbage in the gut helps clean the blood in turn.

I take 50 to 200 mg of 5-hydroxytryptophan (5-HTP), which is a serotonin precursor, along with herbs such as cascara daily. I take a product I designed called Neuro-GI Px, one capsule every night. I eat about a teaspoon of flaxseeds in the evening and the morning, by themselves or in a smoothie, along with a cup of warm water first thing in the morning.

———

In closing this chapter, I'd like to reiterate the unique nature of any given person's experience with multiple sclerosis. I don't expect that everyone with MS will employ all the tips and strategies for daily life that I have outlined here. If you have MS, you know yourself and you know your disease. Please choose and use only those tips that you find helpful.

CHAPTER 10

Expect Nothing, Accept Everything

As I sit at my desk on an early-spring day (the time of year we Vermont-ers call mud season), I can't help but reflect on my experiences with MS and all that I've written about in this book. My thoughts keep returning to this theme: Although I've experienced improvement in my symptoms, and my physical signs of this disease—improvements I hope you, your patients, or your loved ones will also experience—my journey hasn't been without bumps. I still have bad days. Some of them are *really* bad. And I want to reassure you that *that's okay*. Just as icier, colder nights cause maple trees to make sweeter syrup, the worst MS attacks can strengthen emotional and psychological resiliency.

A few years ago I unexpectedly found myself overtaken by a condition called transverse myelitis. Transverse myelitis is an acute attack on the spinal cord; it can occur on its own or in conjunction with MS. It can be mild and temporary or result in permanent quadriplegia. And it is fast . . . it's like having an MS attack on overdrive. The symptoms can manifest in a period of several hours. Previous to this episode, I had been doing everything I could to be as healthy as possible: taking all the protocols for neuroinflammation and neuropro-tection with herbs, diet, hormones, and prescription drugs such as Tecfidera (fumarate). But . . . I was bitten by a tick that was carrying the Lyme disease spirochete, and that I speculated triggered the severe attack. That's the unique aspect of MS. Even if you are doing everything "just right," one small event like a tick bite or a flu can make your life different. Really different. This particular attack began following a fun family day tubing down a river with my kids.

The Next Day That Changed My Life

I woke up suddenly that morning, feeling pretty stiff, but I didn't worry about it too much. I went to my office (only a few miles away). One hour later it was very painful to sit down. Two hours later, I decided that I should go home. I limped away from my desk and with the assistance of co-workers walked to my car. I started driving home, but I felt like my legs were getting weaker. On the spot I made a U-turn and chose to drive a few miles in the other direction to the hospital. Even though I had no appointment, I knew I needed to see my neurologist for an urgent checkup.

In the hospital parking lot, I opened my car door and found I could barely walk. Ever so slowly, like a sloth, I walked all the way to the entrance door but found I couldn't go in. I was feeling self-conscious and didn't ask for help. I was only a few feet away from the hospital doors, but traveling those few feet felt impossible. A hospital attendant rushed over and helped me into a wheelchair. My neurologist saw me in his office and told me I needed to be admitted to the hospital. I was given intravenous infusions of prednisone to treat acute transverse myelitis—an inflammation in both sides of one section of my spinal cord that was interrupting the signals my brain was trying to send to the rest of my body. After three days, despite the steroid infusions, new symptoms arose including transient moments of not being able to talk. Four days later I began experiencing sudden surges of high pulse rate. A week after that I developed trouble swallowing.

I had been thinking that getting an IV of a powerful drug at the hospital would fix me up. It turned out to be not nearly so simple. I also developed symptoms of autonomic dysreflexia, a potentially life-threatening medical emergency. And those challenges continue today, as the story of my autonomic dysreflexia continues to unravel even as this book goes to publication.

As the days wore on, in order to avoid scaring our children, Sarika and I decided not to tell them many details about what was happening to me. Still, kids are intuitive. One morning at breakfast, my four-year-old son looked at her and said, "Papa, if he dies, I'll take care of Mama." I, too, was initially concerned I might die; but I certainly couldn't admit this to my vulnerable and impressionable children, nor even Sarika.

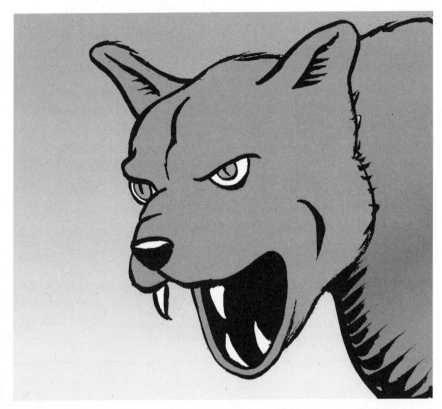

The jaguar that appeared to me in a dream represented the forces beyond my control —those that might leave me seriously disabled, or even kill me. Eventually all MS patients must come to terms with their own "jaguar."

Two weeks before my Lyme-driven attack, I had a vivid dream. I was deep in the forest, aware that a jaguar was gently licking my face. Transfixed and scared, I watched as the huge cat stopped its licking—not to clamp its jaws around one of my limbs, or to devour me whole as I expected—but to regard me with a peaceful expression. I knew that I had to surrender—perhaps even to being eaten.

Behind the powerful jaguar, a woman I didn't recognize explained that all forms in the universe change. The big cat may eat me, or take one of my limbs, or it may simply make a friendly visit—but the jaguar will always come, and come back. After I woke up, I realized that the jaguar represented

---

Autonomic Dysreflexia
(Medical Emergency Card)

Autonomic dysreflexia (AD) results from a sudden rise in blood pressure in an individual with a spinal cord injury (SCI), with a neurological level of T6 or above.

The cause of AD is a pain stimulus below the level of injury, resulting in an unopposed sympathetic system discharge. Raising the blood pressure 20–40 mm Hg systolic above the person's normal baseline blood pressure may trigger the symptoms of AD.

Symptoms of Autonomic Dysreflexia

- Increased blood pressure
- Severe headache
- Flushing and sweating above the level of the SCI
- Bradycardia

- Anxiety
- Cardiac irregularities
- Bronchospasm or respiratory distress
- Goose bumps on the skin above the level of the SCI

If left untreated, this condition can result in seizure, retinal hemorrhage, stroke, or in extreme cases death.

This is my second medical wallet card, more serious than the first. I have had two episodes so far during which my blood pressure shot up 50 points in one hour as a result of autonomic dysreflexia.

my disease and its persistent, raw threat to my identity and body. At any time, the jaguar could revert to its predator nature and inflict physical harm, and there was nothing I could do to prevent that.

Six weeks after the start of that terrible attack of autonomic dysreflexia, I was walking fine. But I still had cardiac problems; I would experience a racing heart and sudden surges of blood pressure.

My doctor recommended an autonomic dysreflexia card to carry with me.

Receiving this card was far more of an emotional blow than when I was given a wallet card for aphasia. An autonomic dysreflexia card is most often given to people who are paraplegic or quadriplegic. Fortunately, I am neither of those. The Christopher Reeve Foundation (founded by the late movie actor who portrayed Superman and who became quadriplegic after a horse-riding accident) is a great resource for anyone who needs or wants more information and support regarding how to live with autonomic dysfunction.

One-third of those who experience transverse myelitis fully recover and return to normal within two years, but because of my MS, my future was uncertain. Some time ago my doctor had told me that a lesion located in my upper cervical spine "could be a ticking time bomb." I had forgotten about it, but now I was reminded of it every day. My inner voice raised questions. *Will this be the moment when I end up in a wheelchair permanently? Will I require full-time assistance with daily activities, even the ones I've prided myself on creating adaptive strategies to handle? What about the book I'm writing? I should be an inspiration to others.* At the end of the day, though, all the "should this" and "should that"s don't get anyone anywhere.

Just a few months before that attack, I had been feeling healthy and confident. We were so relieved that we confidently began planning an epic, monthlong trip to India to visit relatives. The whole immediate family, including my mother-in-law, would go along. We prepared and anticipated and, as the departure date drew closer and closer, our collective excitement shot higher and higher.

By now, you may already have guessed what happened: We didn't go. Instead, we dealt with the crisis and adjusted to a new normal. A year later I was better, and we had allowed ourselves to look forward to the trip we had postponed and rescheduled. In the midst of writing and polishing this chapter, however, I had to make the choice—once again—to cancel the big trip to visit family in India.

Just a few nights before the flight for our rescheduled trip was supposed to depart, I began choking on my own saliva. Rapidly, my symptoms progressed. My heart raced. I had the sensation that it was difficult to inflate my lungs with air (this was due to an innervation issue to the diaphragm). I had difficulty getting enough air, a condition called vocal cord abduction, in which my vocal folds closed up during breathing and obstructed my airway. The effects of my autonomic dysreflexia had returned.

When I was in medical school, I heard the expression that doctors "entertain" the patient while the body does the healing. I can tell you one thing: these "-ologists" did entertain me very well, as they explained the story of why I felt the way I did. One neurologist said they thought what I was experiencing was due to an MS attack at my brain stem. Another neurologist said it was

About Autonomic Dysfunction

Autonomic dysfunction, or autonomic neuropathy, occurs when something causes the autonomic (involuntary) nervous system (ANS) to stop working properly. ANS dysfunction is often a side effect of a specific disease or condition, including MS. Symptoms include:[1]

Postural hypotension, which can cause dizziness, fainting, an unsteady gait, weakness, and other problems.
Urinary dysfunction, including frequency (especially at night), stress incontinence, and retention.
Gastrointestinal problems, including diarrhea, constipation, bloating, nausea, vomiting, appetite loss, and more.
Numbness, especially in the extremities.

In fact, ANS dysfunction can affect almost any of the body's involuntary functions, including heart rate, blood pressure, respiration, body temperature, and digestion. Treatments include addressing the underlying cause(s), and/or managing specific symptoms.

because MS was causing a spinal cord injury. Yet another neurologist thought it was primary autonomic dysfunction that resulted from a Lyme-triggered MS attack on my autonomic system. As I write this, two years following that attack, my neurologist no longer thinks it was caused by MS.

Regardless of the cause, the outcome is that my autonomic dysreflexia has become my "secret job"—one I never applied for, and one I certainly don't want. I have to consciously think about swallowing and managing bladder, bowel, and heart functions on a daily basis—about every three hours or so—which means I can no longer work full-time at my real job. As my autonomic neurologist told me, "There is no pill for this." As I mentioned in the introduction, his declaration struck me as the perfect name for my book.

I was also prescribed Ocrevus, a new drug. Initially, I was very cautious and suspicious of taking this drug, because its mechanism of action is basically to attack the body's own immune system. Taking Ocrevus was not an easy choice. Before it's administered (via IV), you have to sign a disclaimer to hold harmless the hospital, drug manufacturer, and so on, because Ocrevus can increase risk of cancer, fatal brain infection, and other serious issues. Yikes.

Taking Ocrevus reminded me of a science-fiction movie. I sat in a chair and, through the IV tube attached to my arm, I received an antibody that is cloned to attack a certain type of "problematic" white blood cell found in most autoimmune diseases. Out of trillions of cells to attack, the antibody knows to select one type of cell with one type of receptor: a B cell of a certain age. Within six weeks of the treatment, my energy returned, cognitive function normalized, numbness and tingling went away, and my legs collapsed less often. But it never really helped my autonomic dysreflexia, which is by far my most debilitating symptom.

Lessons Learned

My experiences with transverse myelitis and autonomic dysfunction are the two most recent events in my MS journey, and they are among my most intense, too. From them, and, indeed from my whole experience living with MS, this is what I have learned:

Every experience has a silver lining. And a corollary to that: If you can't see the silver lining right away, it's possible to reframe your mindset and create one for yourself.

Here's what I mean.

When I was battling the effects of transverse myelitis, life was very rough. The only way I could get around the house the first night was to lie on the floor and drag myself by the arms, grabbing the walls and the legs of chairs just to move from one part of a room to the next. I felt like an infant who'd just learned to crawl, but the experience carried none of the joy, or celebration, that normally accompanies those sorts of milestones. I'd regressed, not progressed, and my family was sad and scared as they watched me struggle.

Both my father and my brother had been accomplished ice climbers during their lives—in fact, my brother died in an ice climbing accident. And at some point, it struck me that my challenges in getting around the house on the floor were somewhat similar to their accomplishment in climbing a peak. In some ways, it might have been equally satisfying. So with that attitude adjustment, I prepared to traverse the north face of our kitchen.

During this tough time, I felt a sense of significant accomplishment whenever I successfully solved the mental and physical puzzle of getting from point A to point B. I began to appreciate what I *could* do, not what I *couldn't* do—and felt, in many ways, that my horizontal "ice climbing" might even have been more difficult than the vertical kind because I had no choice. For me, the silver lining—the one I'll return to again and again—is that during my struggle to navigate my home, I experienced many pleasant memories of my father and brother that I might otherwise not have recalled. Like the time my brother taught me to climb to the ceiling by pressing both my hands and feet into opposite sides of a doorframe and shimmying to the top.

Within two days after my doctor finally diagnosed me with transverse myelitis, I was tremendously fortunate to regain use of my legs. Still, many other challenges remained. I still couldn't swallow well, for example, and my voice had degenerated to such an extent that it sounded like Stephen Hawking's voice at times. It took many more weeks of intensive therapy to recover, including having to practice enunciating simple sounds like *t* and *z* over and over again. *Honestly* I felt disheartened—especially since my four-year-old daughter was learning to say four-syllable words at the same time—but instead I brought my focus back to my ice-climbing lesson. We shouldn't compare our accomplishments with those of others and make that the basis of our satisfaction. For some people with MS, relearning to walk at age 50 might bring similar satisfaction to that of first learning to walk as a child. If you can walk upright, no matter what your circumstances, you can find satisfaction in that.

Finding, or creating, your own silver lining—while it isn't always easy—is helpful.

I am never fully in control of anything. Despite all of my experiences over the years, it still never ceases to surprise and amaze me how quickly my body and cognition can change. MS has a way of humbling me—reminding me, after each attack, that my ability to pilot the plane of my own future is an illusion.

After all, I took all the right conventional and herbal medicines. I made sure to get enough sleep. I exercised as much as I could. I drank power smoothies. I underwent a fecal transplant and follow-up therapies. I didn't smoke or do drugs. The Indian side of my family teaches that our fate is a partnership between us and God; I was doing my job as I believed it to be, and casting the rest of my fate to a higher power.

In many ways, I did great. Over an eight-year period, the lesion my neurologist had described as a "ticking time bomb" grew very little. But as I aged, my body had more difficulty adjusting to the lesion, and I began experiencing attacks that I couldn't predict and had no way of warding off—despite everything that I was doing right. And no two attacks were exactly the same. Sometimes I'd have balance issues. Other times I couldn't walk. More than once, I couldn't remember simple things like what day it was. My worst underlying fear was that I might not emerge from one of these attacks—that the disability would be permanent. But as I came to understand that I would manage to return to mostly normal function after these attacks, I also came to realize that control is a myth. God may or may not control my fate, but *I* certainly don't. In so many instances when I thought I was in charge, and when I thought I could predict the future, MS smacked me back down to Earth. Planning that trip to India—and assuming I'd be able to go—is the perfect example of this hard-learned lesson.

I work hard every day to focus on not dwelling on my future or when or if my next attack will occur, how bad it might be, and whether I will still be able enjoy and appreciate life with Sarika and our children. I can take pride in accomplishing daily goals, no matter how small. I can acknowledge the sweetness, and preciousness, of everything around me.

I think back to my transverse myelitis, or I remind myself of my current autonomic dysfunction, and remind myself that another attack could very easily happen again—maybe even tomorrow. I'm grateful for what I have right in that moment: another way to actively search for life's silver linings.

I should not take anything for granted. Transverse myelitis taught me that one day I might be running around having fun with my kids, and the next I might be unable to walk. Autonomic dysfunction taught me that one day I could be conversing freely with family and friends, and the next I might have to relearn how to pronounce the letters of the alphabet.

With each attack, I discover something new, about my body and how it reacts and also about the assumptions I have taken for granted: my ability to clearly communicate, to walk, to tie my own shoes, to understand the question someone just asked. Before we had to cancel our first trip to India, I also assumed I'd be able to continue fulfilling my passion for global travel and adventure. Now I'm not entirely sure about that. (But how's this for another silver lining? I've been reminding myself that MS is, in itself, a daily adventure with no known destination!)

I've been extremely fortunate to have recovered from each major setback. But—since I know I have no control over the future—there's no guarantee that I will bounce back the next time, or the time after that. Not taking things for granted is a companion to my humble attempt at a living-in-the-moment philosophy. Every step I take is a gift.

I'm more than my body. At the end of the day, if you think life is great only if all your body parts are functioning well, then life is going to be a big disappointment! I've learned that my spirit, my faith, and my consciousness can bring me contentment more effectively than any treatment or drug can.

As someone who initially considered going to divinity school instead of medical school, I've been inspired, over the years, to explore what some call *renunciation*: the abandonment of physical or material comforts in order to achieve spiritual insights, to live a more "holy" life (whatever that may mean for you), or to experience a higher form of consciousness free from the constraints of having too many choices and distractions that impede what's important in life. Most traditions, from Christianity to Buddhism, include at least some form of the idea of limiting what you can do in order to achieve a higher purpose.

Limiting yourself in life might be freeing. Feeling pain and discomfort while spending time in isolation in meditation or fasting is not necessarily pleasant in the way eating candy is. But life isn't candy, either; and anyway, candy is bad for the microbiome.

In my case, my autonomic dysfunction forced me into feats of strength I wish I *hadn't* had to participate in. I've learned that the best way I can survive my symptoms and manage their challenging effects is to gently try to remember that I might need to renounce what I want, and remember that my consciousness is bigger than myself and my wants.

Thanks to the expert advice from all those "-ologists," and to the strategies I've described in this book, during my worst days, even as I struggled with the very real and very human fear of my own mortality and became frustrated with my limitations, I reminded myself that things wouldn't always be that way. I've learned this lesson again and again with each new attack. It's important not to catastrophize your experience. Life goes on. You need to adapt to the world. The world doesn't adapt to your illness and it shouldn't. The things I've written about in this chapter, perhaps more than anything else in this book, are concrete proof of that. My hope for you is that during *your* worst days—or the worst days of your loved one—you can return to these ideas and find your own comfort and peace.

I did recover from my own worst days. And while I'm never truly the same person I was before an attack—MS has a habit of leaving psychic as well as physical footprints—I want to reiterate that I attribute such ongoing recoveries to the lifestyle modifications I've made as I've learned about this disease.

You see, 10 years ago, when I was first diagnosed with MS, doctors told me my case was "moderate" to "advanced," based on the total number of lesions visible on my MRI. My first MS neurologist told me he had never encountered another patient who already had so many lesions upon first diagnosis. Six years later my second MS neurologist noticed that I no longer had visible cerebral cortical atrophy—the loss of neurons and the connections between them that's characteristic of many neurodegenerative diseases. She also saw that my progression was incredibly slow, with barely any new lesions on an MRI. She called this remarkable, asked me what I was doing, and told me that pharmaceutical drugs alone couldn't explain my results.

I *do* still experience symptoms, and as my third neurologist predicted, even if MS progresses very slowly, the clinical manifestations can be severe. My last attack was due to only a slight growth of a lesion, but in one of the worst areas—a cervical lesion in the autonomic nervous system. Interestingly enough, it was such a small change that the radiology department at a university hospital didn't notice it on the MRI. But MS lesions are like real estate. It's about location, location, location. Now I have a new set of symptoms to manage, and the MS adventure continues.

I have done the best I can and will continue to do so, as best I can. Even with MS, my health is as robust as it can be thanks to natural medicine and the other approaches I've described here. The overall lesson that MS has taught me is that we *can* make choices about our lives; we *can* prioritize where we put our energy and focus. On some days, we will have very few options to choose from, because the body ultimately says *no*. But even then, the mind is always free to choose a path within any limits the body imposes. If you only had 10 steps to take (because your legs don't work well), where would you go? If you only had 20 words to speak (because your throat muscles don't work), what would you say—and to whom?

Multiple sclerosis forces you to prioritize what's really important, and that's the silver lining to the fact that there is no pill for this. Just like when I started this book, MS is an adventure, and we never really know what our future is.

And so I initially set out to prove my doctor was wrong. I was going to find the holy grail. I refused to write myself into a script with only one story line: that everyone with MS gets worse. I never found the holy grail, and I did get worse. Nonetheless, I don't think it means I failed; despite MS attacking my identity I still feel whole and well much of the time.

Whatever curveball MS throws you, please try to do whatever you can, not only to treat your body, but also to accept it. We are on this journey of life (and MS) together. I wish you and your loved ones all the courage and inspiration you need to feel whole.

Frequently Asked Questions

What is MS?

Multiple sclerosis, or MS, is an autoimmune disease of the central nervous system, or CNS. In MS, the body's immune system attacks the myelin sheath, a fatty layer that surrounds and insulates nerve fibers. When the myelin sheath is damaged, messages sent through the CNS are altered or stopped completely.

The word *sclerosis* means "scar tissue." When the myelin sheath is damaged, scar tissue forms. This scar tissue usually appears in multiple places. Thus the name *multiple sclerosis*.

What is myelin?

Myelin is an insulating layer of fat and protein that forms around nerves. Myelin functions similarly to the plastic insulation on an electrical wire. When the myelin sheath is healthy, the nerves conduct impulses rapidly and send accurate signals. When the myelin sheath is damaged, as it is in multiple sclerosis, nerve impulses slow down or stop. These "short circuits" in the nervous system cause a variety of neurological symptoms.

What are the symptoms of MS?

For people with MS, symptoms vary widely. They can include symptoms that come and go, and symptoms that become progressively worse over time. The most common symptoms include:

- Vision problems
- Cognitive problems

- Depression
- Difficulty walking
- Tingling and numbness
- Pains, spasms, and itching
- Weakness and fatigue
- Bladder or bowel issues
- Dizziness and vertigo
- Sexual problems

What causes MS?

The cause of MS is unknown. Researchers believe it may be linked to genetics, environmental factors, bacteria or viruses, low levels of vitamin D_3, and abnormalities in the immune system. Recent research explores a possible link between MS and leaky gut syndrome. In this condition, diet and other factors create an imbalance in the trillions of bacteria and other organisms that inhabit the human gut. This imbalance causes inflammation that damages the gut's protective lining, allowing toxins to leak from the gut. Some of these toxins can breach the gut-brain barrier and enter the brain and spinal cord, where they do damage to myelin.

Does CCSVI cause MS?

In 2009 Italian physician and researcher Dr. Paolo Zamboni did a study in which he noticed that the veins leading back toward the heart from the brain and spinal cord appeared constricted in people with MS. This constriction is known as chronic cerebrospinal venous insufficiency or CCSVI. Zamboni theorized that CCSVI caused blood pressure to rise in the brain and spinal cord, leading to inflammation and causing MS. He theorized that venous angioplasty to remove constriction from the veins in the neck might relieve MS symptoms.

Unfortunately, studies of Dr. Zamboni's theories have shown no evidence that CCSVI causes MS or that treatment for CCSVI can relieve MS symptoms. In 2017 a clinical trial with over 100 patients showed that venous angioplasty in people with MS had no effect on their disease. And as of early 2020, studies showed no conclusive link between CCSVI and MS. Although CCSVI does not necessarily correlate with causation, I have heard of enough patients (including my medical doctor) who have been so improved by the treatment that I still consider CCSVI as a possible effective treatment for MS (but not a cure).

How is MS diagnosed?

There is no single test to confirm that a person has multiple sclerosis. Diagnosis can be difficult and take time. Doctors weigh a number of factors. They look at physical, cognitive, and emotional symptoms. They usually do an MRI to look for the characteristic scarring or plaques formed by damage to myelin in the brain and spinal cord. They may also tap spinal fluid and analyze the fluid for antibodies associated with MS. At the same time, they work to rule out other diseases that could cause symptoms similar to those the patient is experiencing. One way to do this is through blood tests.

Can MS be cured?

At present, there is no cure for MS, but various treatments have been shown to slow its progress or reduce the frequency and severity of outbreaks. Western treatment regimens include corticosteroids to reduce nerve inflammation, beta interferon, and pharmaceuticals including ocrelizumab (Ocrevus), glatiramer acetate, and many others. Restorative and naturopathic treatments include following a diet to reduce inflammation and alter the human microbiome, fecal microbiome transplants, herbs, supplements, hormones, exercise, yoga, and meditation.

How common is MS?

According to the National MS Society, about one-tenth of 1 percent of Americans are at risk for developing MS. In general, people living farther from the equator tend to be more likely to develop the disease. Caucasians of Northern European ancestry have the highest risk of getting MS. It is less common in other groups, including people of African, Latino, and Asian origin. Some populations of people, including the Inuit people, Norwegian Lapps, Hutterites, and Aboriginal Australians, virtually never get the disease. MS is four times more prevalent in women than men, although men usually have a poorer prognosis.

What are the different types of MS?

There are three types of MS:

Relapsing-remitting MS (RRMS). Up to 80 percent of people with MS have this type, making it by far the most common. In RRMS people experience periods called flare-ups, relapses, or exacerbations during which symptoms are evident. Relapses usually last a day to a few weeks. During periods known as remission, the symptoms seem to disappear, but the disease is still present and can progress.

Secondary progressive MS (SPMS). In this type of MS, symptoms worsen over time. People with SPMS may experience periods of relapse and remission as well, although not all people with SPMS do. Many people with RMSS progress to SPMS over time.

Primary progressive MS (PPMS). In this type of MS, the disease slowly worsens over time without relapse or remission. PPMS affects about 10 percent of people with MS.

In chapter 1 of this book, I also mention a fourth type, clinically isolated syndrome, which is a single episode of neurological symptoms that are suggestive of MS. Some people never progress beyond this episode, but others go on to develop one of the above types of MS.

What supplements/drugs do I take every day?

1. Bacopa extract
2. Green tea extract
3. Thymosin beta-4 daily injection
4. Rosmarinic Acid* (made with high dose of rosmarinic acid and quercetin)
5. Neuro-Protect* (made with lion's mane and ashwagandha extracts)
6. Enfla-Mend* (made with turmeric extract and turmeric essential oils / turmerones)
7. MicroBiome* (goldenseal/berberine product)
8. Mitochondrial Nutrition PQQ* daily multi with vitamin D₃ and PQQ
9. Neuro-GI* (triphala, cascara, and 5-HTP)

---

* These are all products I designed for my company Restorative Formulations.

Can children get MS?

While it is uncommon, children and teens can get MS. Young people develop only relapsing-remitting MS, or RRMS. Early symptoms can manifest as fatigue, learning disorders, and clumsiness.

Is MS genetic?

Studies and statistics on people with MS seem to indicate that there is a genetic component. In identical twins, for example, if one twin develops MS, the other twin will develop it about 25 percent of the time. This is a much higher incidence than in the general population. The higher incidence of MS in Caucasians and the lower incidence or virtual nonexistence of it in certain populations seem to support the idea of a genetic link.

Is there a link between MS and smoking?

Definitely. According to the National Multiple Sclerosis Society, people who smoke are more likely to contract MS. People with MS who smoke will progress to secondary progressive MS at a faster rate, and have greater risk of increasing disability. Quitting smoking now will reduce the risk of contracting MS. And if you have already been diagnosed with MS, quitting smoking can slow the progression of your disease.

What is the link between MS and depression?

Depression is one of the most common symptoms of MS. People with MS are more likely to experience depression than people in the general population. It's important to know that depression can make other symptoms such as pain and fatigue seem worse. It's also important to know that people can't just "cheer up" and wish their depression away. Depression is, however, treatable by a mental health professional. If depression is present, treatment for it should be part of an MS care plan.

Does MS shorten life expectancy?

People with MS tend to have a shorter life span than the general population. One study showed that they tend to die 6 to 10 years earlier than people in the general population. The disease itself is responsible for the majority of earlier deaths, but death rates from some other causes, including suicide, heart disease, and infection, are higher for people with MS as well.

Can vitamin K be helpful in treating MS?

While new research into vitamin K is promising, scientists don't know what role the vitamin plays in MS and what role it might play in treatment. Vitamin K helps regulate calcium storage, bone metabolism, and blood clotting. It may play a role in reducing inflammation. A recent study has shown that people with MS have much lower vitamin K levels than people without MS. The reason why is unclear. It may be that lower vitamin K levels play a role in causing MS—or that these lower levels are a result of MS. Further studies will be needed to understand vitamin K's role in MS and its use as a possible treatment.

Can bee sting therapy reduce MS symptoms?

Many people have promoted and tried the use of bee sting therapy to activate the immune system and ease MS symptoms. While bee venom therapy has been shown to be safe—except, of course for people with allergies to bee venom—there is no evidence that it provides any help for people with MS.

Can fecal implants reduce the symptoms of MS?

Fecal microbial transplantation, or FMT, is a process by which a fecal preparation from a healthy donor is transplanted into the colon of a patient who is sick with a disease. The theory behind FMT is that an imbalance in microbes in a person's gut can cause or contribute to some diseases, and that a fecal transplant can restore a healthy balance of microbes and ease the symptoms of those diseases. FMT has been used successfully to treat infection with recurrent *Clostridium difficile*, a type of bacteria that infects the digestive tract and causes chronic diarrhea and damage to the intestinal tract. Because researchers have noted a connection between imbalance in the microbiome and MS, they have begun experimenting with fecal transplants. Some early results, including FMT transplants performed at the Taymount Clinic, have shown promise in reducing symptoms but not decreasing progression of the illness. Studies are under way to further investigate the possibility of using FMT to treat MS.

Why are people with MS prone to UTIs?

Urinary tract infections (UTIs) occur when bacteria enter the urinary tract and grow there, causing symptoms ranging from pain and urinary urgency to fever and fatigue. People with MS often have difficulty fully emptying their bladder. The urine left behind can provide a place for bacteria to grow. Using a catheter can help people with MS to fully empty the bladder. But using a catheter increases risk that bacteria will be introduced into the urinary tract, causing infection. Commonly, UTIs are treated with antibiotics, but they can recur.

To avoid UTIs, drink plenty of water, avoid constipation, and use good personal hygiene. Women should be careful to wipe from front to back to avoid contamination of the urinary tract with fecal bacteria.

Notes

Introduction

1. Brandi Koskie, "Multiple Sclerosis: Facts, Statistics, and You," *Healthline*, last modified June 20, 2018, http://www.healthline.com/health/multiple-sclerosis/facts-statistics-infographic.

2. Koskie, "Multiple Sclerosis."

Chapter 1: Driving on the Wrong Side of the Road

1. "Types of MS," National Multiple Sclerosis Society, accessed May 13, 2020, https://www.nationalmssociety.org/What-is-MS/Types-of-MS.

2. Howard Weiner, "Multiple Sclerosis: The History of a Disease," *New England Journal of Medicine* 2005, no. 353 (September 2005): 1306–07, http://doi.org/10.1056/NEJMbkrev38300.

3. Zawn Villines, "How Does Dawson's Finger Relate to Multiple Sclerosis?" *Medical News Today*, updated May 20, 2019, https://www.medicalnewstoday.com/articles/315437.php.

Chapter 2: The Ones Who Leave the Jungle

1. F. Coperchini et al., "Thyroid Disruption by Perfluorooctane Sulfonate (PFOS) and Perfluorooctanoate (PFOA)," *Journal of Endocrinological Investigation* 40, no. 2 (February 2017): 105–21; "Common Flame Retardant Chemical Disrupts a Hormone That Is Essential to Life," Endocrine Society, April 2, 2016, https://www.endocrine.org/news-and-advocacy/news-room/2016/common-flame-retardant-chemical-disrupts-a-hormone-that-is-essential-to-life.

2. Manivannan Yegambaram et al., "Role of Environmental Contaminants in the Etiology of Alzheimer's Disease: A Review," *Current Alzheimer Research* 12, no. 2 (February 2015): 116–46, http://doi.org/10.2174/1567205012666150204121719.

3. Julie Gardham, "Book of the Month, October 2003," review of *Pathological Anatomy: Illustrations of the Elementary Forms of Disease*, by Robert Carswell, October 2003, http://special.lib.gla.ac.uk/exhibns/month/oct2003.html.

4. "The 4 Types of MS," Multiple Sclerosis (MS): Better Questions Lead to Better Answers, Bayer, accessed May 13, 2020, https://www.multiplesclerosis.com/us/treatment.php.

5. "Cognitive Changes," National Multiple Sclerosis Society, accessed May 13, 2020, https://www.nationalmssociety.org/Symptoms-Diagnosis/MS-Symptoms/Cognitive-Changes.

6. Anthony Feinstein and Bennis Pavisian, "Mutiple Sclerosis and Suicide," *Multiple Sclerosis* 23, no. 7 (June 2017): 923–27, http://doi.org/10.1177/1352458517702553.

7. Marjaleena Koskiniemi et al., "Piracetam Relieves Symptoms in Progressive Myoclonus Epilepsy: A Multicentre, Randomised, Double Blind, Crossover Study Comparing the Efficacy and Safety of Three Dosages of Oral Piracetam with Placebo," *Journal of Neurology, Neurosurgery and Psychiatry* 64, no. 3 (March 1998): 344–48, http://doi.org/10.1136/jnnp.64.3.344.

8. T. Wagemans et al., "Clinical Efficacy of Piracetam in Cognitive Impairment: A Meta-Analysis," *Dementia and Geriatric Cognitive Disorder* 13 (2002): 2017–24, http://doi.org/10.1159/000057700.

Chapter 3: A Loss of Balance

1. David Perlmutter and Kristin Loberg, *Grain Brain: The Surprising Truth about Wheat, Carbs, and Sugar—Your Brain's Silent Killers* (London: Yellow Kite, 2019), 28.

2. Yun Kyung Lee et al., "Proinflammatory T-Cell Responses to Gut Microbiota Promote Experimental Autoimmune Encephalomyelitis," *Proceedings of the National Academy of Sciences of the United States of America* 108, supplemental 1 (March 2011): 4615–22, http://doi.org/10.1073/pnas.1000082107.

3. Lee et al., "Proinflammatory T-Cell Responses," 4615–22.

4. Paolo Riccio and Rocco Rossano, "Nutrition Facts in Multiple Sclerosis," *ASN Neuro* 7, no. 1 (February 18, 2015): 1–20, http://doi.org/10.1177/1759091414568185.

5. Giulia-Anna Perri, "Complications of End-Stage Liver Disease," *Canadian Family Physician* 61, no. 1 (January 2016): 44–50.

6. Donald McNeil, Jr., "Deadly, Drug-Resistant 'Superbugs' Pose Huge Threat, WHO Says," *New York Times*, February 27, 2017, https://www.nytimes.com/2017/02/27/health/who-bacteria-pathogens-antibiotic-resistant-superbugs.html.

7. L. Dethlefsen et al., "The Pervasive Effects of an Antibiotic on the Human Gut Microbiota, as Revealed by Deep 16S rRNA Sequencing," *PLoS Biology* 6, no. 11 (November 2008): 2383–400.

8. Ilseung Cho et al., "Antibiotics in Early Life Alter the Murine Colonic Microbiome and Adiposity," *Nature* 488 (2012): 621–26; Laura Cox et al., "Altering the Intestinal Microbiota during a Critical Developmental Window Has Lasting Metabolic Consequences," *Cell* 158, no. 4 (August 2014): 705–21.

9. Aaron Lerner et al., "The World Incidence and Prevalence of Autoimmune Disease Is Increasing," *International Journal of Celiac Disease* 3, no. 4 (July 2018), 151–55.

10. Shilpa Ravella, "How the Food You Eat Affects Your Gut," *TEDEd*, accessed May 13, 2020, https://ed.ted.com/lessons/how-the-food-you-eat-affects-your-gut-shilpa-ravella.

11. Alessio Fasano, "Zonulin and Its Regulation of Intestinal Barrier Function: The Biological Door to Inflammation, Autoimmunity, and Cancer," *Physiological Reviews* 91, no. 1 (January 2011): 151–75, http://doi.org/10.1152/physrev.00003.2008.

12. Riccio and Rossano, "Nutrition Facts in Multiple Sclerosis," 1–20.

13. K. Hillman et al., "Colonization of the Gastric Contents of Critically Ill Patients," *Critical Care Medicine* 10, no. 7 (July 1982): 444–47.

14. Damon DiSabato, Ning Quan, and Jonathan Godbout, "Neuroinflammation: The Devil Is in the Details," *Journal of Neurochemistry* 139, supplemental 2 (October 2016): 136–53, http://doi.org/10.1111/jnc.13607.

15. Renée F. A. G. de Bruijn and M. Arfan Ikram, "Cardiovascular Risk Factors and Future Risk of Alzheimer's Disease," *BMC Medicine* 12 (November 2014): 130, http://doi.org /10.1186/s12916-014-0130-5.

16. Nancy Lane et al., "Tanezumab for the Treatment of Pain from Osteoarthritis of the Knee," *New England Journal of Medicine* 363 (2010): 1521–31, http://doi.org/10.1056 /NEJMoa0901510.

17. Stephen Skaper et al., "An Inflammation-Centric View of Neurological Disease: Beyond the Neuron," *Frontiers in Cellular Neuroscience* 12 (March 2018): 72, http://doi.org /10.3389/fncel.2018.00072.

18. Fabrizia Monteleone et al., "Nerve Growth Factor Is Elevated in the CSF of Patients with Multiple Sclerosis and Central Neuropathic Pain," *Journal of Neuroimmunology* 314 (January 2018): 89–93, http://doi.org/10.1016/j.jneuroim.2017.11.012.

19. Luisa Bracci-Laudiero et al., "Multiple Sclerosis Patients Express Increased Level of β-Nerve Growth Factor in Cerebrospinal Fluid," *Neuroscience Letters* 147, no. 1 (December 1992): 9–12, http://doi.org/10.1016/0304-3940(92)90762-V.

20. Eric Wohleb et al., "β-Adrenergic Receptor Antagonism Prevents Anxiety-Like Behavior and Microglial Reactivity Induced by Repeated Social Defeat," *Journal of Neuroscience* 31, no.17 (April 2011): 6277–88, http://doi.org/ 10.1523/JNEUROSCI.0450-11.2011.

21. DiSabato, Quan, and Godbout, "Neuroinflammation: The Devil Is in the Details," 136–53.

22. Roshni A. Desai et al., "Cause and Prevention of Demyelination in a Model Multiple Sclerosis Lesion," *Annals of Neurology* 79, no. 4 (April 2016): 591–604, http://doi.org /10.1002/ana.24607.

23. Paul Eggleton et al., "Manipulation of Oxygen and Endoplasmic Reticulum Stress Factors as Possible Interventions for Treatment of Multiple Sclerosis: Evidence for and Against," *Multiple Sclerosis: Bench to Bedside* (January 2017): 11–27, http://doi.org/10.1007/978-3 -319-47861-6_2.

24. E. Shokri-Kojori et al., "β-Amyloid Accumulation in the Human Brain after One Night of Sleep Deprivation," *Proceedings of the National Academy of Science, United States* 115, no. 7 (April 2018): 4483–88, http://doi.org/10.1073/pnas.1721694115.

25. Giovanna De Chiara et al., "Infectious Agents and Neurodegeneration," *Molecular Neurobiology* 46, no. 3 (December 2012): 614–38, http://doi.org/10.1007/s12035-012-8320-7.

26. Roisin M. McManus and Michael Heneka, "Role of Neuroinflammation in Neurodegeneration: New Insights," *Alzheimer's Research and Therapy* 9, no. 1 (March 2017): 14, http://doi.org/10.1186/s13195-017-0241-2.

27. McManus and Heneka, "Role of Neuroinflammation," 14.

28. Stephen Blackmore et al., "Influenza Infection Triggers Disease in a Genetic Model of Experimental Autoimmune Encephalomyelitis," *Proceedings of the National Academy of Science, United States* 114, no. 30 (July 2015): E6107–16, http://doi.org/10.1073/pnas .1620415114.

29. McManus and Heneka, "Role of Neuroinflammation," 14.

30. Jacques De Keyser, Cornelis Zwanikken, and Maartje Boon, "Effects of Influenza Vaccination and Influenza Illness on Exacerbations in Multiple Sclerosis," *Journal of the Neurological Sciences* 159, no. 1 (July 1998): 51–53, http://doi.org/10.1016/S0022 -510X(98)00139-7.

31. DiSabato, Quan, and Godbout, "Neuroinflammation: The Devil Is in the Details," 136–53.

32. Kim Ohl, Klaus Tenbrock, and Markus Kipp, "Oxidative Stress in Multiple Sclerosis: Central and Peripheral Mode of Action, *Experimental Neurology* 277 (March 2016): 58–67, http://doi.org/10.1016/j.expneurol.2015.11.010.

33. Ohl, Tenbrock, and Kipp, "Oxidative Stress," 58–67.

34. Maxime Jeanjean et al., "Short-Term Exposure to Ambient Air Pollution and Occurrence of Multiple Sclerosis Relapses" (poster, ECTRIMS Online Library, October 2017), https://onlinelibrary.ectrims-congress.eu/ectrims/2017/ACTRIMS-ECTRIMS 2017/200145/maxime.jeanjean.short-term.exposure.to.ambient.air.pollution.and .occurrence.of.html.

35. Emeran Mayer, Kirsten Tillisch, and Arpana Gupta, "Gut/Brain Axis and the Microbiota," *Journal of Clinical Investigation* 125, no. 3 (March 2015): 926–38, http://doi.org/10.1172 /JCI76304.

36. Staffan Holqvist et al., "Direct Evidence of Parkinson Pathology Spread from the Gastrointestinal Tract to the Brain in Rats," *Acta Neuropathologica* 128, no. 6 (December 2014): http://doi.org/10.1007/s00401-014-1343-6.

37. Rashad Alkasir et al., "Human Gut Microbiota: The Links with Dementia Development," *Protein and Cell* 8, no. 2 (February 2017): 90–102, http://doi.org/10.1007/s13238-016 -0338-6.

38. James Hill et al., "Pathogenic Microbes, the Microbiome, and Alzheimer's Disease (AD)," *Frontiers in Aging Neuroscience* 6 (June 2014): 127, http://doi.org/10.3389/fnagi.2014 .00127.

39. Hill et al., "Pathogenic Microbes," 127.

40. Melanie Gareau, "Microbiota-Gut-Brain Axis and Cognitive Function," *Advances in Experimental Medicine and Biology* 817 (June 2014): 357–71, http://doi.org/10.1007/978-1 -4939-0897-4_16.

41. W. N. Marks et al., "The Effect of Chronic Corticosterone on Fear Learning and Memory Depends on Dose and the Testing Protocol," *Neuroscience* (March 2015): 324–33, http:// doi.org/10.1016/j.neuroscience.2015.01.011.

42. Katarina Raduolovic et al., "Interjections of Lipopolysaccharide into Mice to Mimic Entrance of Microbial-Derived Products after Intestinal Barrier Breach," *Journal of Visual Experiments* no. 128 (May 2018): http://doi.org/10.3791/57610; Miryam Nava Catorce and Goar Gevorkian, "LPS-Induced Murine Neuroinflammation Model: Main Features and Sustainability for Pre-Clinical Assessment of Nutraceuticals," *Current Neuropharmacology* 14, no. 2 (February 2016): 155–64, http://doi.org/10.2174/1570159X146661 51204122017.

43. Alessio Fasano, "Zonulin and Its Regulation of Intestinal Barrier Function: The Biological Door to Inflammation, Autoimmunity, and Cancer," *Physiology Review* 91, no. 1 (January 2011): 151–75, http://doi.org/10.1152/physrev.00003.2008.

44. Maarten Witte et al., "Mitochondrial Dysfunction Contributes to Neurodegeneration in Multiple Sclerosis," *Trends in Molecular Medicine* 20, no. 3 (March 2014): 179–87, http:// doi.org/10.1016/j.molmed.2013.11.007.

Chapter 4: Returning to the Jungle

1. Thomas Borody et al., "Fecal Microbiota Transplantation (FMT) in Multiple Sclerosis (MS)," *American Journal of Gastroenterology* 106 (October 2011): 106.

2. Mary Jane Brown, "How Short-Chain Fatty Acids Affect Health and Weight," *Healthline*, updated April 2, 2016, https://www.healthline.com/nutrition/short-chain-fatty-acids-101.

3. "High Dietary Fiber Intake Linked to Health Promoting Short Chain Fatty Acids: Beneficial Effects Not Limited to Vegetarian or Vegan Diets," *ScienceDaily*, updated September 29, 2015, https://www.sciencedaily.com/releases/2015/09/150929070122.htm.

Chapter 5: Putting Out the Fire of Neuroinflammation

1. L. J. Spielman, J. P. Little, and A. Klegeris, "Physical Activity and Exercise Attenuate Neuroinflammation in Neurological Diseases," *Brain Research Bulletin* 125 (July 2016): 19–29, http://doi.org/10.1016/j.brainresbull.2016.03.012.

2. Spielman, Little, and Klegeris, "Physical Activity," 19–29.

3. Spielman, Little, and Klegeris, "Physical Activity," 19–29.

4. Gwenn Smith, "Aging and Neuroplasticity," *Dialogues in Clinical Neuroscience* 15, no. 1 (March 2013): 3–5, https://www.ncbi.nlm.nih.gov/pmc/articles/PMC3622467.

5. G. M. Petzinger et al., "Exercise-Enhanced Neuroplasticity Targeting Motor and Cognitive Circuitry in Parkinson's Disease," *Lancet Neurology* 12, no. 7 (July 2013): 716–26, http://doi.org/ 10.1016/S1474-4422(13)70123-6.

6. N. Preisler et al., "Effect of Aerobic Training in Patients with Spinal and Bulbar Muscular Atrophy (Kennedy Disease)," *Neurology* 72, no. 4 (January 2009): 317–23, http://doi.org/10.1212/01.wnl.0000341274.61236.02.

7. "Canadian Physical Activity Guidelines," Canadian Society for Exercise Physiology (CSEP), accessed May 14, 2020, http://www.csep.ca/CMFiles/Guidelines/specialpops/CSEP_MS_PAGuidelines_adults_en.pdf.

8. Mary Harmon, "Exercise as Part of Everyday Life" (National Multiple Sclerosis Society, 2016), https://www.nationalmssociety.org/NationalMSSociety/media/MSNationalFiles/Brochures/Brochure-Exercise-as-Part-of-Everyday-Life.pdf.

9. "How Much Is Too Much?" SugarScience, University of California–San Francisco, accessed May 14, 2020, http://sugarscience.ucsf.edu/the-growing-concern-of-overconsumption.html#.W8yLGmhKhPY.

10. "How Much Is Too Much?"

11. Mariangela Farinotti et al., "Dietary Interventions for Multiple Sclerosis," *Cochrane Database Systematic Review* no. 12 (December 2012): http://doi.org/10.1002/14651858.CD004192.pub3.

12. Chia-Yu Chang, Der-Shin Ke, and Jen-Yin Chen, "Essential Fatty Acids and Human Brain," *Acta Neurologica Taiwanica* 18, no. 4 (December 2009): 231–41.

13. Welayah Ali AlAmmar et al., "Effect of Omega-3 Fatty Acids and Fish Oil Supplementation on Multiple Sclerosis: A Systematic Review," *Nutritional Neuroscience* (August 2019): 1–11, http://doi.org/10.1080/1028415X.2019.1659560; Julie Stachowiak, "Omega-3 Fatty Acids for Multiple Sclerosis," *Very Well Health*, updated April 13, 2020, https://www.verywellhealth.com/omega-3-fatty-acids-and-multiple-sclerosis-2440487.

14. S. C. Dyall and A. T. Michael-Titus, "Neurological Benefits of Omega-3 Fatty Acids," *Neuromolecular Medicine* 10, no. 4 (2008): 219–35, http://doi.org/10.1007/s12017-008-8036-z.

15. Cecilia Samieri et al., "Plasma Long-Chain Omega-3 Fatty Acids and Atrophy of the Medial Temporal Lobe," *Neurology* 79, no. 7 (August 2012): 642–50, http://doi.org/10.1212/WNL.0b013e318264e394.

16. Pao-Yen Lin et al., "A Meta-Analytic Review of Polyunsaturated Fatty Acid Compositions in Dementia," *Journal of Clinical Psychiatry* 73, no. 9 (August 2012): 1245–54, http://doi.org10.4088/JCP.11r07546.

17. Steven Brenner, "Red Blood Cell Omega-3 Fatty Acid Levels and Markers of Accelerated Brain Aging," *Neurology* 79, no. 1 (July 2012): 106–07, http://doi.org/10.1212/WNL.0b013e31825e41b2.

18. Ji Yeon Choi et al., "Antarctic Krill Oil Diet Protects against Lipopolysaccharide-Induced Oxidative Stress, Neuroinflammation and Cognitive Impairment," *International Journal of Molecular Sciences* 18, no. 12 (November 2017): 2554, http://doi.org/10.3390/ijms18122554.

19. Mikhail Shchepinov, Mark Mattson, and Brian Bennett, "A New Treatment Paradigm for Neurodegeneration: Peroxidation-Resistant Polyunsaturated Fatty Acids (D-PUFA) Lower Brain Amyloid Beta and Oxidation Markers, and Reverse Cognition Impairment in Vivo (P4.090)," *Neurology* 88, supplemental 16 (April 2017).

20. Paul Boston et al., "Ethyl-EPA in Alzheimer's Disease—A Pilot Study," *Prostaglandins, Leukotrienes and Essential Fatty Acids* 71, no. 5 (November 2004): 341–46, http://doi.org/10.1016/j.plefa.2004.07.001; Joseph Quinn et al., "Docosahexaenoic Acid Supplementation and Cognitive Decline in Alzheimer Disease: A Randomized Trial," *JAMA* 304, no. 17: 1903–11, http://doi.org/10.1001/jama.2010.1510.

21. L. K. Lee et al., "Docosahexaenoic Acid-Concentrated Fish Oil Supplementation in Subjects with Mild Cognitive Impairment (MCI): A 12-Month Randomised, Double-Blind, Placebo-Controlled Trial," *Psychopharmacology* 225, no. 3 (August 2012): 605–12, http://doi.org/10.1007/s00213-012-2848-0; Dyall and Michael-Titus, "Neurological Benefits of Omega-3 Fatty Acids," 219–35.

22. Vijayshree Yadav et al., "Summary of Evidence-Based Guideline: Complementary and Alternative Medicine in Multiple Sclerosis: Report of the Guideline Development Subcommittee of the American Academy of Neurology," *Neurology* 82, no. 12 (March 2014): 1083–92, http://doi.org/10.1212/WNL.0000000000000250.

23. E. J. Hadgkiss et al., "The Association of Diet with Quality of Life, Disability, and Relapse Rate in an International Sample of People with Multiple Sclerosis," *Nutritional Neuroscience* 18, no 3 (April 2015): 125–36, http://doi.org/10.1179/1476830514Y.0000000117.

24. Vijayshree Yadav et al., "Low-Fat, Plant-Based Diet in Multiple Sclerosis: A Randomized Controlled Trial," *Multiple Sclerosis and Related Diseases* 9 (September 2016): 80–90, http://doi.org/10.1016/j.msard.2016.07.001.

25. Ilana Katz Sand, "The Role of Diet in Multiple Sclerosis: Mechanistic Connections and Current Evidence," *Current Nutrition Reports* 7, no. 3 (August 2018): 150–60, http://doi.org/10.1007/s13668-018-0236-z.

26. Yadav et al., "Low-Fat, Plant-Based Diet in Multiple Sclerosis," 80–90.

27. Carl E. Stafstrom and Jong Rho, eds., *Epilepsy and the Ketogenic Diet* (Totowa, NJ: Humana Press, 2004).

28. Terry L. Wahls, "Wahls Paleo Diet and Progressive Multiple Sclerosis," *Clinical Trials*, updated June 26, 2018, https://clinicaltrials.gov/ct2/show/NCT01915433.

29. R. L. Swank, "Treatment of Multiple Sclerosis with Low-Fat Diet: Results of Five and One-Half Years' Experience," *AMA Archives of Neurology and Psychiatry* 73, no. 6 (1955): 631–44, http://doi.org/10.1001/archneurpsyc.1955.02330120035004.

30. T. Wahls et al., "Dietary Approaches to Treat MS-Related Fatigue: Comparing the Modified Paleolithic (Wahls Elimination) and Low Saturated Fat (Swank) Diets on Perceived Fatigue in Persons with Relapsing-Remitting Multiple Sclerosis: Study Protocol for a Randomized Control Trial," *Trials* 19, no. 1 (June 2018): 309, http://doi.org/10.1186/s13063-018-2680-x.

31. Morena Martucci et al., "Mediterranean Diet and Inflammaging within the Hormesis Paradigm," *Nutrition Reviews* 75, no. 5 (June 2017): 442–55, http://doi.org/10.1093/nutrit/nux013.

32. Rajagopal Sekhar, "Glutathione in Mild Cognitive Impairment" (study record, Clinical-Trials.gov, US National Library of Medicine, updated December 17, 2019), https://clinicaltrials.gov/ct2/show/NCT03493178.

33. Christina Hoffmann et al., "Dimethyl Fumarate Induces Glutathione Recycling by Upregulation of Glutathione Reductase," *Oxidative Medicine and Cellular Longevity* 2017 (January 2017): 1–8, http://doi.org/10.1155/2017/6093903.

34. Roberto Bomprezzi, "Dimethyl Fumarate in the Treatment of Relapsing-Remitting Multiple Sclerosis: An Overview," *Therapeutic Advances in Neurological Disorders* 8, no. 1 (January 2015): 20–30, http://dio.org/10.1177/1756285614564152.

35. Emanuela Eposito et al., "Fumaric Acid Esters as a New Therapeutic Target for Traumatic Brain Injury," *FASEB Journal* 31, supplemental 1 (April 2017): 815.1.

36. Mythily Srinivasana and Debomoy Lahiri, "Significance of NF-κB as a Pivotal Therapeutic Target in the Neurodegenerative Pathologies of Alzheimer's Disease and Multiple Sclerosis," *Expert Opinion on Therapeutic Targets* 19, no. 4 (March 2018): 471–87, http://doi.org/10.1517/14728222.2014.989834.

37. Srinivasana and Lahiri, "Significance of NF-κB," 471–87.

38. Patrick Griffin and Esther Care, eds., *Assessment and Teaching of 21st Century Skills: Methods and Approach* (Dordrecht, Netherlands: Springer, 2015).

39. Joost Schulte and J. Troy Littleton, "The Biological Function of the Huntingtin Protein and Its Relevance to Huntington's Disease Pathology," *Current Trends in Neurology* 5 (January 2011): 65–78, https://www.ncbi.nlm.nih.gov/pmc/articles/PMC3237673.

40. Sivagami Giridharan and Mythily Srinivasan, "Mechanisms of NF-κB p65 and Strategies for Therapeutic Manipulation," *Journal of Inflammation Research* 11 (October 2018): 407–19, http://doi.org/10.2147/JIR.S140188.

41. Heba Ghaiad et al., "Resveratrol Promotes Remyelination in Cuprizone Model of Multiple Sclerosis: Biochemical and Histological Study," *Molecular Neurobiology* 54 (2017): 3219–29, http://doi.org/10.1007/s12035-016-9891-5.

42. Shatadal Ghosh, Sharmistha Banerjee, and Parames C. Sil, "The Beneficial Role of Curcumin on Inflammation, Diabetes and Neurodegenerative Disease: A Recent Update," *Food and Chemical Toxicology* 83 (September 2015): 111–24, http://doi.org/10.1016/j.fct.2015.05.022.

43. "Turmeric: Curcuma Longa 1," Association for the Advancement of Restorative Medicine, https://restorativemedicine.org/library/monographs/turmeric-1/#sd endnote48sym.

44. Bahare Salehi et al., "The Therapeutic Potential of Curcumin: A Review of Clinical Trials," *European Journal of Medicinal Chemistry* 163 (February 2019): 527–45, http://doi .org/10.1016/j.ejmech.2018.12.016.

45. Shusuke Toden and Ajay Goel, "The Holy Grail of Curcumin and Its Efficacy in Various Diseases: Is Bioavailability Truly a Big Concern?" *Journal of Restorative Medicine* 6, no. 1 (December 2017): 27–36.

46. Silvia Rossi, Giorgio Bernardi, and Diego Centonze, "The Endocannabinoid System in the Inflammatory and Neurodegenerative Process of Multiple Sclerosis and of Amyotrophic Lateral Sclerosis," *Experimental Neurology* 224, no. 1 (July 2010): 92–102, http://doi.org/10.1016/j.expneurol.2010.03.030.

Chapter 6: Reinsulating the Wires

1. Nancy Lane et al., "Tanezumab for the Treatment of Pain from Osteoarthritis of the Knee," *New England Journal of Medicine* 363, no. 16 (October 2010): 1521–31, http://doi .org/10.1056/NEJMoa0901510.

2. Fabrizia Monteleone et al., "Nerve Growth Factor Is Elevated in the CSF of Patients with Multiple Sclerosis and Central Neuropathic Pain," *Journal of Neuroimmunology* 314 (January 2018): 89–93, http://doi.org/10.1016/j.jneuroim.2017.11.012.

3. Stephen Skaper et al., "An Inflammation-Centric View of Neurological Disease: Beyond the Neuron," *Frontiers in Cellular Neuroscience* 12 (March 2018): 72, http://doi.org/10.3389 /fncel.2018.00072.

4. Kevin Spelman, Elizabeth Sutherland, and Aravind Bagade, "Neurological Activity of Lion's Mane (*Hericium eranaceus*)," *Journal of Restorative Medicine* 6 (2017): 19–26, http:// doi.org/10.14200/jrm.2017.6.0108.

5. Spelman, Sutherland, and Bagade, "Neurological Activity of Lion's Mane," 19–26.

6. Calliandra Harris et al., "Dietary Pyrroloquinoline Quinone (PQQ) Alters Indicators of Inflammation and Mitochondrial-Related Metabolism in Human Subjects," *Journal of Nutritional Biochemistry* 24, no. 12 (December 2013): 2076–84, http://doi.org/10.1016 /j.jnutbio.2013.07.008.

7. Kohji Yamaguchi et al., "Stimulation of Nerve Growth Factor Production by Pyrroloquin- oline Quinone and Its Derivatives in Vitro and in Vivo," *Bioscience, Biotechnology, and Biochemistry* 57, no. 7 (February 1993): 1231–33, http://doi.org/10.1271/bbb.57.1231.

8. Hirokatsu Takatsu et al., "Effect of Vitamin E on Learning and Memory Deficit in Aged Rats," *Journal of Nutritional Science and Vitaminology* 55, no. 5 (October 2009): 389–93, http://doi.org/10.3177/jnsv.55.389.

9. Lili Zhang et al., "The Neuroprotective Effect of Pyrroloquinoline Quinone on Traumatic Brain Injury," *Journal of Neurotrauma* 29, no. 5 (March 2012): 851–64, http://doi.org/10 .1089/neu.2011.1882.

10. Frédéric Sedel et al., "Targeting Demyelination and Virtual Hypoxia with High-Dose Biotin as a Treatment for Progressive Multiple Sclerosis," *Neuropharmacology* 110, part B (November 2016): 644–53, http://doi.org/10.1016/j.neuropharm.2015.08.028.

11. "Biotin: Fact Sheet for Health Professionals," Office of Dietary Supplements, National Institutes of Health, updated July 9, 2019, https://ods.od.nih.gov/factsheets/Biotin -HealthProfessional.

12. Frédéric Sedel et al., "High Doses of Biotin in Chronic Progressive Multiple Sclerosis: A Pilot Study," *Multiple Sclerosis and Related Disorders* 4, no. 2 (March 2015): 159–69, http:// doi.org/10.1016/j.msard.2015.01.005.

13. Ayman Tourbah et al., "MD1003 (High-Dose Biotin) for the Treatment of Progressive Multiple Sclerosis: A Randomised, Double-Blind, Placebo-Controlled Study," *Multiple Sclerosis* 22, no. 13 (September 2016): 1719–31, http://doi.org/10.1177/1352458516667568.

14. Ayman Tourbah et al., "Effect of MD1003 (High Doses of Biotin) in Chronic Visual Loss Related to Optic Neuritis in Multiple Sclerosis (MS-ON): Results of a Pivotal Randomized Double Masked Placebo Controlled Study (S49.005)," *Neurology* 86, supplemental 16 (April 2016); Ayman Tourbah et al., "MD1003 (High-Dose Pharmaceutical-Grade Biotin) for the Treatment of Chronic Visual Loss Related to Optic Neuritis in Multiple Sclerosis: A Randomized, Double-Blind, Placebo-Controlled Study," *CNS Drugs* 32, no. 7 (July 2018): 661–72, http://doi.org/10.1007/s40263-018-0528-2.

15. Arthur Warrington, "High Dose Biotin, MD1003, Protects Axons in a Mouse Model of Chronic Spinal Cord Demyelination (P2.2-057)," *Neurology* 92, supplemental 15 (April 2019).

16. F. Granella et al., "Breakthrough Disease under High-Dose Biotin Treatment in Progressive Multiple Sclerosis," *ECTRIMS Online Library*, updated October 26, 2017, https:// onlinelibrary.ectrims-congress.eu/ectrims/2017/ACTRIMS-ECTRIMS2017/200405/ franco.granella.breakthrough.disease.under.high-dose.biotin.treatment.in.html.

17. "The FDA Warns That Biotin May Interfere with Lab Tests: FDA Safety Communication," FDA, updated November 5, 2019, https://www.fda.gov/medical-devices/safety -communications/fda-warns-biotin-may-interfere-lab-tests-fda-safety-communication.

Chapter 7: Regulating the Regulators

1. "Neuroendocrine System," *Science Direct*, accessed May 15, 2020, https://www.science direct.com/topics/agricultural-and-biological-sciences/neuroendocrine-system.

2. Yasuhiro Nishiyama and Ken-Ichiro Katsura, "The Neuroendocrine System and Its Regulation," in *Neuroanesthesia and Cerebrospinal Protection*, ed. Hiroyuki Uchino, Kazuo Ushijima, and Yukio Ikeda (Tokyo: Springer, 2015), 31–38, http://doi.org/10.1007 /978-4-431-54490-6_3.

3. Natalie Ebner et al., "Hormones as 'Difference Makers' in Cognitive and Socioemotional Aging Processes," *Frontiers in Psychology* 5 (January 2015): 1595, http://doi.org/10.3389 /fpsyg.2014.01595; T. E. Seeman and B. S. McEwen, "Impact of Social Environment Characteristics on Neuroendocrine Regulation," *Psychosomatic Medicine* 58, no. 5 (1996): 459–71, http://doi.org/10.1097/00006842-199609000-00008.

4. Anne Cappola, Qian-Li Xue, and Linda Fried, "Multiple Hormonal Deficiencies in Anabolic Hormones Are Found in Frail Older Women: The Women's Health and Aging Studies," *Journals of Gerontology* 64A, no. 2 (February 2009): 243–48, http://doi.org /10.1093/gerona/gln026.

5. Nan Wang et al., "Effects of Thyroxin and Donepezil on Hippocampal Acetylcholine Content and Syntaxin-1 and Munc-18 Expression in Adult Rats with Hypothyroidism,"

Experimental and Therapeutic Medicine 7, no. 3 (March 2014): 529–36, http://doi.org /10.3892/etm.2014.1487.

6. Mao Zhang et al., "Thyroid Hormone Potentially Benefits Multiple Sclerosis via Facilitating Remyelination," *Molecular Neurobiology* 53 (September 2016): 4406–16, http://doi .org/10.1007/s12035-015-9375-z.

7. Borja Belandia et al., "Thyroid Hormone Negatively Regulates the Transcriptional Activity of the Beta-Amyloid Precursor Protein Gene," *Journal of Biological Chemistry* 273, no. 46 (November 1998): 30366–71, http://doi.org/10.1074/jbc.273.46.30366.

8. John Walsh et al., "Subclinical Thyroid Dysfunction as a Risk Factor for Cardiovascular Disease," *Archives of Internal Medicine* 165, no. 21 (2005): 2467–72, http://doi.org/10 .1001/archinte.165.21.2467.

9. Zaldy Tan et al., "Thyroid Function and the Risk of Alzheimer's Disease: The Framingham Study," *Archives of Internal Medicine* 168, no. 14 (July 2008): 1514–20, http://doi.org /10.1001/archinte.168.14.1514.

10. J. S. Solka et al., "Co-Occurrence of Autoimmune Thyroid Disease in a Multiple Sclerosis Cohort," *Journal of Autoimmune Disease* 2, no. 1 (December 2005): 9, http://doi.org/10 .1186/1740-2557-2-9.

11. C. Brian Bai et al., "A Mouse Model for Testing Remyelinating Therapies," *Experimental Neurology* 283, part A (September 2016): 330–40, http://doi.org/10.1016/j.expneurol .2016.06.033; Mao Zhang et al., "Thyroid Hormone Alleviates Demyelination Induced by Cuprizone through Its Role in Remyelination during the Remission Period," *Experimental Biology and Medicine* 240, no. 9 (September 2015): 1183–96, http://doi.org /10.1177/1535370214565975.

12. Markus Kipp et al., "Thalamus Pathology in Multiple Sclerosis: From Biology to Clinical Application," *Cellular and Molecular Life Science* 72 (2015): 1127–47, http://10.1007/s00018 -014-1787-9.

13. Dwayne K. Hamson, Meighen M. Roes, and Liisa A. M. Galea, "Sex Hormones and Cognition: Neuroendocrine Influences on Memory and Learning," *Comprehensive Physiology* 6, no. 3 (July 2016): 1295–337, http://doi.org/10.1002/cphy.c150031.

14. Rhonda Voskuhl and Callene Momtazee, "Pregnancy: Effect on Multiple Sclerosis, Treatment Considerations, and Breastfeeding," *Neurotherapeutics* 14, no. 4 (October 2017): 974–84, http://doi.org/10.1007/s13311-017-0562-7.

15. Claudia Barth, Arno Villringer, and Julia Sacher, "Sex Horomones Affect Neurotransmitters and Shape the Adult Female Brain during Hormonal Transition Periods," *Frontiers in Neuroscience* 9, no. 37 (2015): 37, http://doi.org/10.3389/fnins.2015.00037.

16. Natalie C. Ebner et al., "Hormones as 'Difference Makers' in Cognitive and Socioemotional Aging Processes," *Frontiers in Psychology* 5, (January 2015), https://doi.org/10.3389 /fpsyg.2014.01595.

17. Pauline M. Maki and Victor W. Henderson, "Hormone Therapy, Dementia, and Cognition: The Women's Health Initiative 10 Years On," *Climacteric* 15, no. 3 (June 2012): 256–62, http://doi.org/10.3109/13697137.2012.660613.

18. Seema Tiwari-Woodruff and Rhonda R. Voskuhl, "Neuroprotective and Anti-Inflammatory Effects of Estrogen Receptor Ligand Treatment in Mice," *Journal of Neurological Sciences* 286, no. 1–2 (November 2009): 81–85, http://doi.org/10.1016/j.jns.2009.04.023;

S. Kim at al., "Estriol Ameliorates Autoimmune Demyelinating Disease: Implications for Multiple Sclerosis," *Neurology* 52, no. 6 (April 1999): 1230–38, http://doi.org/10.1212/WNL.52.6.1230.

19. Rhonda R. Voskuhl et al., "Estriol Combined with Glatiramer Acetate for Women with Relapsing-Remitting Multiple Sclerosis: A Randomised, Placebo-Controlled, Phase 2 Trial," *Lancet Neurology* 15, no. 1 (January 2016): 35–36, http://doi.org/10.1016/S1474-4422(15)00322-1.

20. M. A. Hernan et al., "Oral Contraceptives and the Incidence of Multiple Sclerosis," *Neurology* 55, no. 6 (September 2000): 848–54, http://doi.org/10.1212/WNL.55.6.848.

21. Jane Marjoribanks et al., "Long-Term Hormone Therapy for Perimenopausal and Postmenopausal Women," *Cochrane Database of Systematic Reviews* no. 1 (2017): CD004143, http://doi.org/10.1002/14651858.CD004143.pub5.

22. Bushra Imtiaz et al., "Risk of Alzheimer's Disease among Users of Postmenopausal Hormone Therapy: A Nationwide Case-Control Study," *Maturitas* 98 (April 2017): 7–13, http://doi.org/10.1016/j.maturitas.2017.01.002.

23. Maki and Henderson, "Hormone Therapy, Dementia, and Cognition," 256–62.

24. Kejal Kantarcia et al., "Early Postmenopausal Transdermal 17β-Estradiol Therapy and Amyloid-β Deposition," *Journal of Alzheimer's Disease* 53, no. 2 (July 2016): 547–56, http://doi.org/10.3233/JAD-160258.

25. Michael Schumacher et al., "Progesterone Synthesis in the Nervous System: Implications for Myelination and Myelin Repair," *Frontiers in Neuroscience* 6 (2012): 10, http://doi.org/10.3389/fnins.2012.00010.

26. M. Meyer et al., "Protective Effects of the Neurosteroid Allopregnanolone in a Mouse Model of Spontaneous Motoneuron Degeneration," *Journal of Steroid Biochemistry and Molecular Biology* 174 (November 2017): 201–16, http://doi.org/10.1016/j.jsbmb.2017.09.015.

27. Schumacher et al., "Progesterone Synthesis in the Nervous System," 10.

28. Emily R. Rosario and Christian J. Pike, "Androgen Regulation of β-Amyloid Protein and the Risk of Alzheimer's Disease," *Brain Research Reviews* 57, no. 2 (March 2008): 444–53, http://doi.org/10.1016/j.brainresrev.2007.04.012.

29. Shima Tavakol et al., "Self-Assembling Peptide Nanofiber Containing Long Motif of Laminin Induces Neural Differentiation, Tubulin Polymerization, and Neurogenesis: In Vitro, ex Vivo, and in Vivo Studies," *Molecular Neurobiology* 53, no. 8 (October 2016): 5288–99, http://doi.org/10.1007/s12035-015-9448-z.

30. Rosario and Pike, "Androgen Regulation of β-Amyloid Protein," 444–53.

31. S. Giatti et al., "Dihydrotestosterone as a Protective Agent in Chronic Experimental Autoimmune Encephalomyelitis," *Neuroendocrinology* 101 (2015): 296–308, http://doi.org/10.1159/000381064.

32. J. Holland, S. Bandelow, and E. Hogervorst, "Testosterone Levels and Cognition in Elderly Men: A Review," *Maturitas* 69, no. 4 (August 2011): 322–37, http://doi.org/10.1016/j.maturitas.2011.05.012.

33. M. M. Cherrier et al., "Testosterone Improves Spatial Memory in Men with Alzheimer Disease and Mild Cognitive Impairment," *Neurology* 64, no. 12 (June 2005): 2063–68, http://doi.org/10.1212/01.WNL.0000165995.98986.F1; Po Lu et al., "Effects of Testosterone on Cognition and Mood in Male Patients with Mild Alzheimer Disease and

Healthy Elderly Men," *Archives of Neurology* 63, no. 2 (2006): 177–85, http://doi.org /10.1001/archneur.63.2.nct50002.

34. Terrell T. Gibbs, Shelley J. Russek, and David H. Farb, "Sulfated Steroids as Endogenous Neuromodulators," *Pharmacology Biochemistry and Behavior* 84, no. 4 (August 2006): 555–67, http://doi.org/10.1016/j.pbb.2006.07.031.

35. Patrizia Porcu et al., "Neurosteroidogenesis Today: Novel Targets for Neuroactive Steroid Synthesis and Action and Their Relevance for Translational Research," *Journal of Neuroendocrinology* 28, no. 2 (February 2016), https://doi.org/10.1111/jne.12351.

36. Tangui Maurice, Catherine Gregoire, and Julie Espallergues, "Neuro(active)steroids Actions at the Neuromodulatory Sigma$_1$ (σ_1) Receptor: Biochemical and Physiological Evidences, Consequences in Neuroprotection," *Pharmacology Biochemistry and Behavior* 84, no. 4 (August 2006): 581–97, http://doi.org/10.1016/j.pbb.2006.07.009.

37. Sebastien Weill-Engerer et al., "Neurosteroid Quantification in Human Brain Regions: Comparison between Alzheimer's and Nondemented Patients," *Journal of Clinical Endocrinology and Metabolism* 87, no. 11 (November 2002): 5138–43, http://doi.org/10.1210 /jc.2002-020878.

38. H. Meziane et al., "The Neurosteroid Pregnenolone Sulfate Reduces Learning Deficits Induced by Scopolamine and Has Promnestic Effects in Mice Performing an Appetitive Learning Task," *Psychopharmacology* 125 (August 1996): 323–30, http://doi.org/10.1007 /BF02247383.

39. Natalie C. Ebner et al., "Hormones as 'Difference Makers' in Cognitive and Socioemotional Aging Processes," *Frontiers in Psychology* 5 (January 2015): 1595, http://doi.org /10.3389/fpsyg.2014.01595.

40. S. Chetty et al., "Stress and Glucocorticoids Promote Oligodendrogenesis in the Adult Hippocampus," *Molecular Psychiatry* 19 (December 2014): 1275–83, http://doi.org /10.1038/mp.2013.190.

41. Christian Otte et al., "A Meta-Analysis of Cortisol Response to Challenge in Human Aging: Importance of Gender," *Psychoneuroendocrinology* 30, no. 1 (December 2004): 80–91, http://doi.org/10.1016/j.psyneuen.2004.06.002.

42. Y. F. Chen et al., "Neuropsychiatric Disorders and Cognitive Dysfunction in Patients with Cushing's Disease," *Chinese Journal of Medicine* 126, no. 16 (August 2013): 3156–60.

43. Sherwood E. Brown et al., "Hippocampal Volume, Spectroscopy, Cognition, and Mood in Patients Receiving Corticosteroid Therapy," *Biological Psychiatry* 55, no. 5 (2004): 538–45, http://doi.org/10.1016/j.biopsych.2003.09.010.

44. S. J. Lupien et al., "The Effects of Stress and Stress Hormones on Human Cognition: Implications for the Field of Brain and Cognition," *Brain and Cognition* 65, no. 3 (December 2007): 209–37, http://doi.org/10.1016/j.bandc.2007.02.007.

45. Mauricio F. Farez et al., "Anti-Inflammatory Effects of Melatonin in Multiple Sclerosis," *Bioessays* 38, no. 10 (August 2016): http://doi.org/10.1002/bies.201600018.

46. Farez et al., "Anti-Inflammatory Effects of Melatonin."

47. M. Adamczyk-Sowa et al., "Influence of Melatonin Supplementation on Serum Antioxidative Properties and Impact of the Quality of Life in Multiple Sclerosis Patients," *Journal of Physiological Pharmacology* 65, no. 4 (August 2014): 453–50, https://www.ncbi .nlm.nih.gov/pubmed/25179086.

48. Mauricio F. Farez et al., "Melatonin Contributes to the Seasonality of Multiple Sclerosis Relapse," *Cell* 162, no. 6 (September 2015): 1338–52, http://doi.org/10.1016/j.cell .2015.08.025.

49. Adamczyk-Sowa et al., "Influence of Melatonin Supplementation on Serum Antioxidative Properties," 453–50.

Chapter 8: The Great Communicators

1. Veronica Francardo et al., "Neuroprotection and Neurorestoration as Experimental Therapeutics for Parkinson's Disease," *Experimental Neurology* 298, part B (December 2017): 137–47, http://doi.org/10.1016/j.expneurol.2017.10.001.

2. Jolanta Dorszewska et al., "Chapter 10: Serotonin in Neurological Diseases," in *Serotonin: A Chemical Messenger between All Types of Living Cells*, ed. Kaneez Fatima Shad (InTech, 2017), http://www.intechopen.com/books/serotonin-a-chemical-messenger-between -all-types-of-living-cells.

3. Gwenn S. Smith et al., "Molecular Imaging of Serotonin Degeneration in Mild Cognitive Impairment," *Neurobiology of Disease* 105 (September 2017): 33, http://doi.org/10.1016/j .nbd.2017.05.007.

4. Michael Messaoudi et al., "Assessment of Psychotropic-Like Properties of a Probiotic Formulation (*Lactobacillus helveticus* R0052 and *Bifidobacterium longum* R0175) in Rats and Human Subjects," *British Journal of Nutrition* 105, no. 5 (March 2011): 755–64, http:// doi.org/10.1017/S0007114510004319.

5. "Gut Microbiome May Modify Neurodegeneration," Society for Neuroscience Annual Meeting 2017, posted December 22, 2017, https://www.alzforum.org/news/conference -coverage/gut-microbiome-may-modify-neurodegeneration; Lap Ho et al., "Protective Roles of Intestinal Microbiota Derived Short Chain Fatty Acids in Alzheimer's Disease– Type Beta-Amyloid Neuropathological Mechanisms," *Expert Review of Neurotherapeutics* 18, no. 1 (January 2018): 83–90, http://doi.org/10.1080/14737175.2018.1400909.

6. Tingting Zhang et al., "Association between the Use of Selective Serotonin Reuptake Inhibitors and Multiple Sclerosis Disability Progression," *Pharmacoepidemiology and Drug Safety* 25, no. 10 (October 2016): 1150–59, http://doi.org/10.1002/pds.4031.

7. Jop P. Mostert et al., "Fluoxetine Increases Cerebral White Matter NAA/Cr Ratio in Patients with Multiple Sclerosis," *Neurosciense Letters* 402, nos. 1–2 (July 2006): 22–24, http://doi.org/10.1016/j.neulet.2006.03.042; Igor Allaman et al., "Fluoxetine Regulates the Expression of Neurotrophic/Growth Factors and Glucose Metabolism in Astro- cytes," *Psychopharmacology* 216 (2011): 75–84, http://doi.org/10.1007/s00213-011 -2190-y; Ebenezer K. C. Kong, "Up-Regulation of 5-HT2B Receptor Density and Receptor-Mediated Glycogenolysis in Mouse Astrocytes by Long-Term Fluoxetine Administration," *Neurochemical Research* 27 (2002): 113–20, http://doi.org/10.1023 /A:1014862808126.

8. Maria Di Bari et al., "Dysregulated Homeostasis of Acetylcholine Levels in Immune Cells of RR-Multiple Sclerosis Patients," *International Journal of Molecular Sciences* 17, no. 2 (2016): http://doi.org/10.3390/ijms17122009.

9. J. P. Higgins and L. Flicker, "Lecithin for Dementia and Cognitive Impairment," *Cochrane Database of Systematic Reviews* 4 (2000), http://doi.org/10.1002/14651858.CD001015.

10. E. Nurk et al., "Plasma Free Choline, Betaine and Cognitive Performance: The Hordaland Health Study." *British Journal of Nutrition* 109, no. 3 (2013): 511–19, http://doi.org/10.1017/S0007114512001249.

11. C. Poly et al., "The Relation of Dietary Choline to Cognitive Performance and White-Matter Hyperintensity in the Framingham Offspring Cohort," *American Journal of Clinical Nutrition* 94, no. 6 (2011): 1584–91, http://doi.org/10.3945/ajcn.110.008938.

12. A. L. Buchman et al., "Verbal and Visual Memory Improve after Choline Supplementation in Long-Term Total Parenteral Nutrition: A Pilot Study," *Journal of Parenteral and Enteral Nutrition* 25, no. 1 (2001): 30–35, http://doi.org/10.1177/014860710102500130; M. Naber, B. Hommel, and L. S. Colzato, "Improved Human Visuomotor Performance and Pupil Constriction after Choline Supplementation in a Placebo-Controlled Double-Blind Study," *Scientific Reports* 5 (August 14, 2015): 13188, http://doi.org/10.1038/srep13188.

13. E. T. Leermakers et al., "Effects of Choline on Health across the Life Course: A Systematic Review," *Nutrition Reviews* 73, no. 8 (2015): 500–22, http://doi.org/10.1093/nutrit/nuv010.

14. Higgins and Flicker, "Lecithin for Dementia and Cognitive Impairment."

15. Oscar Arias-Carrion et al., "Dopaminergic Reward System: A Short Integrative Review," *International Archives of Medicine* 3 (2010): 24, http://doi.org/10.1186/1755-7682-3-24.

16. J. Kira et al., "Hyperprolactinemia in Multiple Sclerosis," *Journal of the Neurological Sciences* 102, no. 1: 61–66, http://doi.org/10.1016/0022-510x(91)90094-n; Recai Turkoglu et al., "Serum Prolactin Levels in Multiple Sclerosis, Neuromyelistis Optica, and Clinically Isolated Syndrome Patients," *Archives of Neuropsychiatry* 53, no. 4 (December 2016): 353–56, http://doi.org/10.5152/npa.2016.16979.

17. Rodrigo Pacheco, Francisco Contreras, and Moncef Zouali, "The Dopaminergic System in Autoimmune Diseases," *Frontiers in Immunology* 5 (2014): 117, http://doi.org/10.3389/fimmu.2014.00117.

18. Mia Levite, Franca Marino, and Marco Cosentino, "Dopamine, T Cells and Multiple Sclerosis (MS)," *Journal of Neural Transmission* 124, no. 5 (2017): 525–42, http://doi.org/10.1007/s00702-016-1640-4.

19. Levite, Marino, and Cosentino, "Dopamine, T Cells and Multiple Sclerosis (MS)," 525–42.

20. Ekaterina Dobryakova et al., "The Dopamine Imbalance Hypothesis of Fatigue in Multiple Sclerosis and Other Neurological Disorders," *Frontiers in Neurology* 6 (March 2015): 52, http://doi.org/10.3389/fneur.2015.00052.

21. Akinori Akaike et al., "Mechanisms of Neuroprotective Effects of Nicotine and Acetyl-cholinesterase Inhibitors: Role of $\alpha 4$ and $\alpha 7$ Receptors in Neuroprotection," *Journal of Molecular Neuroscience* 40, no. 1–2 (January 2010): 211–16, http://doi.org/10.1007/s12031-009-9236-1.

22. Mauricio O. Nava-Mesa et al., "GABAergic Neurotransmission and New Strategies of Neuromodulation to Compensate Synaptic Dysfunction in Early Stages of Alzheimer's Disease," *Frontiers in Cellular Neuroscience* 8 (2014): 167, http://doi.org/10.3389/fncel.2014.00167.

23. Niamh Cawley et al., "Reduced Gamma-Aminobutyric Acid Concentration Is Associated with Physical Disability in Progressive Multiple Sclerosis," *Brain* 138, no. 9 (September 2015): 2584–95, http://doi.org/10.1093/brain/awv209.

Chapter 9: Managing MS Day-to-Day

1. J. Tamar Kalina, "Clutter Management for Individuals with Multiple Sclerosis," *International Journal of MS Care* 16, no. 3 (Fall 2014): 117–22, http://doi.org/10.7224/1537 -2073.2013-035.

2. Laura Mandolesi et al., "Effects of Physical Exercise on Cognitive Functioning and Wellbeing: Biological and Psychological Benefits," *Frontiers in Psychology* 9 (2018): 509, http://doi.org/10.3389/fpsyg.2018.00509.

3. Fernando Gomez-Pinilla, "The Influences of Diet and Exercise on Mental Health through Hormesis," *Ageing Research Reviews* 7, no. 1 (January 2008): 49–62, http://doi.org/10 .1016/j.arr.2007.04.003.

4. J. S. Volek et al., "Testosterone and Cortisol in Relationship to Dietary Nutrients and Resistance Exercise," *Journal of Applied Physiology* 82, no. 1 (January 1997): 49–54, http://doi.org/10.1152/jappl.1997.82.1.49.

5. Sung-Hyun Park and MinYoung Song, "Effects of Aerobic and Anaerobic Exercise on Spatial Learning Ability in Hypothyroid Rats: A Pilot Study," *Journal of Physical Therapy Science* 28, no. 12 (December 2016): 3489–92, http://doi.org/10.1589/jpts.28.3489.

6. Andrea Doring et al., "Exercise in Multiple Sclerosis—An Integral Component of Disease Management," *EPMA Journal* 3, no. 1 (2012): 2, http://doi.org/10.1007/s13167-011-0136-4.

7. "Exercising for Better Sleep," John Hopkins Medicine, accessed May 16, 2020, https://www.hopkinsmedicine.org/health/wellness-and-prevention/exercising-for-better-sleep.

8. "Blue Light Has a Dark Side," Harvard Health Publishing, updated August 2018, https://www.health.harvard.edu/staying-healthy/blue-light-has-a-dark-side.

9. Scott L. Davis et al., "Thermoregulation in Multiple Sclerosis," *Journal of Applied Physiology* 109, no. 5 (November 2010): 1531–37, http://doi.org/10.1152/japplphysiol.00460.2010.

10. Julie Loebach Wetherell et al., "Mindfulness-Based Stress Reduction for Older Adults with Stress Disorders and Neurocognitive Difficulties: A Randomized Controlled Trial," *Journal of Clinical Psychiatry* 78, no. 7 (July 2017): e734, http://doi.org/10.4088/JCP .16m10947.

11. David C. Mohr et al., "A Randomized Trial of Stress Management for the Prevention of New Brain Lesions in MS," *Neurology* 79, no. 5 (July 2012): 412–19, http://doi.org/10 .1212/WNL.0b013e3182616ff9.

12. David Mohr, "Stress Management for Patients with Multiple Sclerosis" (study report, ClinicalTrials.gov, US National Library of Medicine, updated September 2013), https://clinicaltrials.gov/ct2/show/NCT00147446.

13. Sonia Batista et al., "Disconnection as a Mechanism for Social Cognition Impairment in Multiple Sclerosis," *Neurology* 89, no. 1 (July 2017): http://doi.org/10.1212/WNL .0000000000004060.

14. "Sexual Problems," National Multiple Sclerosis Society, accessed May 16, 2020, https://www.nationalmssociety.org/Symptoms-Diagnosis/MS-Symptoms/Sexual-Dysfunction.

15. "Pregnancy and Reproductive Issues," National Multiple Sclerosis Society, accessed May 16, 2020, https://www.nationalmssociety.org/Living-Well-With-MS/Diet-Exercise -Healthy-Behaviors/Womens-Health/Pregnancy.

16. Patricia Silva, "#CMSC16—Aging MS Patients Experience Greater Physical Dysfunction," *Multiple Sclerosis News Today*, updated June 8, 2016, https://multiplesclerosisnewstoday

.com/news-posts/2016/06/08/older-adults-with-ms-experience-low-age-related
-physical-function.

17. Terry DiLorenzo, "Aging with Multiple Sclerosis" (National Multiple Sclerosis Society,
2011), https://www.nationalmssociety.org/NationalMSSociety/media/MSNational
Files/Brochures/Clinical-Bulletin-Aging.pdf.

18. Nancy Holland and Robin Frames, "Bowel Problems: The Basic Facts" (National Multiple
Sclerosis Society, 2009), https://www.nationalmssociety.org/NationalMSSociety
/media/MSNationalFiles/Brochures/Brochure-Bowel-Problems.pdf.

Chapter 10: Expect Nothing, Accept Everything

1. "Autonomic Neuropathy or Autonomic Dysfunction (Syncope): Information and Instruc-
tions," Cleveland Clinic, updated November 30, 2016, https://my.clevelandclinic.org
/health/diseases/15631-autonomic-neuropathy-or-autonomic-dysfunction-syncope
-information-and-instructions; Christine Case-Lo, "Autonomic Dysfunction," *Healthline*,
updated May 13, 2016, https://www.healthline.com/health/autonomic-dysfunction.

Index

Note: Page numbers in *italics* refer to figures.

About the Author

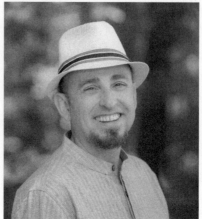

Barrie Fisher Photo

Naturopathic physician Dr. Michaël Friedman is the founder of the Association for the Advancement of Restorative Medicine and the *Journal of Restorative Medicine*. He also creates and formulates herbal and nutritional supplements, and is cofounder and president of the Restorative Formulations supplement company. He is the author of the medical textbook *Fundamentals of Naturopathic Endocrinology*, a contributing author of *Evidence-Based Approach to Restoring Thyroid Health*, and co-author of *Healing Diabetes*. He has treated patients with illnesses ranging from lymphoma to liver cancer, achieving remarkable results that have been published in several medical journals. He lives with his family in Montpelier, Vermont.